# THE
# **SPARK**
# FACTOR

# THE
# SPARK
# FACTOR

### THE SECRET TO SUPERCHARGING ENERGY, BECOMING RESILIENT, AND FEELING BETTER THAN EVER

## Molly Maloof, MD

HARPER WAVE

*An Imprint of HarperCollinsPublishers*

THE SPARK FACTOR. Copyright © 2023 by Molly Maloof. All rights reserved. Printed in the United States of America. No part of this book may be used or reproduced in any manner whatsoever without written permission except in the case of brief quotations embodied in critical articles and reviews. For information, address HarperCollins Publishers, 195 Broadway, New York, NY 10007.

HarperCollins books may be purchased for educational, business, or sales promotional use. For information, please email the Special Markets Department at SPsales@harper collins.com.

FIRST EDITION

Library of Congress Cataloging-in-Publication Data has been applied for.

ISBN 978-0-06-320720-2

23 24 25 26 27  LBC  5 4 3 2 1

I WANT TO DEDICATE THIS BOOK TO MY INCREDIBLE
PARENTS AND MY FOUR SISTERS FOR THEIR UNCONDITIONAL LOVE
THAT HAS HELPED ME UNDERSTAND THE MEANING OF LIFE.

# Contents

# Foreword

Dr. Molly and I met onstage in 2019 as we were participating in a panel on biohacking. The press dubbed me the "Father of Biohacking" because I started the movement more than a decade ago. Today, what was once fringe has gone mainstream—*Merriam-Webster* has even added the word *biohacking* to the dictionary.

I'm forever curious about how far we can upgrade our human hardware and software to extend our capabilities—and even our lifespans—beyond their natural limits. I've spent millions of dollars experimenting with the latest innovations, tools, and techniques that put my body into the maximum longevity zone (which is closer to two hundred years than it is to one hundred years, and possibly a lot more) and increase mental performance and resilience. If somebody out there is biohacking at a high level, I probably know about them.

And yet—I hadn't heard about Dr. Molly Maloof. Who was this new young doctor on the stage next to me? The first thing I noticed about her was her keen mind. I was impressed with how much she knew and (as it turns out) how much younger she looks than she actually is. She was proof of concept! She was biohacking like a pro, and I wondered why I hadn't heard of her before.

At the time, she was working as a concierge doctor in Silicon Valley. She wasn't out promoting herself; she was helping other people improve so they could promote *themselves*. She was consulting for tech companies who were getting all the glory. Meanwhile, she was quietly operating behind the scenes, picking up knowledge like a sponge, teaching students at Stanford how to optimize their health for maximum performance, and putting all the pieces into place so that when she was ready, she could step into the spotlight, with her own company, and with her own book.

That's what she's done now—stepped into the spotlight—and that's exciting. Molly has one of the most open, curious, questioning, and critical sensibilities I've met, and even though she is a biohacking expert, she's always on a quest to learn more, to tackle the next big question, to put into practice the latest discoveries. When I learned she was writing a book, I was thrilled. Most interesting to me was that she had teased apart the differences in how various interventions affect men and women differently. Men are not larger versions of women, and vice versa. And we are all unique, which makes biohacking both an art and a science.

In almost a thousand episodes of *The Human Upgrade* podcast, I've interviewed dozens of women in the biohacking field. Many of the biohacks that work for men work for women too, but there are some disparities. Different hormone profiles require different interventions, and the fluctuating, cyclical nature of female hormones makes biohacking all the more complex and interesting.

What Dr. Molly has done in her groundbreaking book—the first mainstream biohacking book for women that I've seen—is take the tools, principles, and innovations from the sometimes esoteric and inaccessible world of professional, high-level biohacking, and transform them into something people who may never have tried biohacking can understand and engage with. She starts out with a basic but little-understood principle from biohacking: energy powers life. She sheds new light on what's going on inside your body, especially for those who don't remember much from high school biology about mitochondria. This is the spark after which she titled her book: that spark of energy in the cellular batteries that powers your life. Treat your mitochondria right and you treat your body right.

How do you do that? Molly shows you exactly how. Those cellular batteries do so much more than hold a charge, and you'll learn how to charge them, how to use them, and how to really plug them in. One of the coolest things about this book is that, while readers will learn how to biohack their diet and exercise for maximum energetic capacity, *The Spark Factor* also teaches how to combat the draining effects of stress, which is something that runs down everyone's batteries. Molly sheds new light on foundational stress from childhood trauma and "unsafety" signals, as well as all the ways hormones exert themselves in a woman's life (and how to hack them), along with all the stuff about relationships and sex that you were afraid to ask your doctor about. This book is truly a comprehensive guide.

Everyone can learn something here. Whatever it is that interests you about health—your diet, your microbiome, your ideal workout, your sex life, your hormonal transition, your psyche, or your spirituality—Molly can discuss at a high level; she can explain it in easy-to-understand terms; and she can give you a lifestyle prescription to address it, fix it, or take it to the next level. That's a rare skill. Not many genius-level brains belong to warm and approachable people, and she certainly has that "spark" the book talks about—that spark we all seek to capture and harness. She's an innovator, entrepreneur, and a futurist (and it takes one to know one!). I like how her mind works. She sees what's coming, and she has the knowledge to back it up. She consults with many of the most forward-thinking tech companies working for the betterment of human health, so she has the insider information you'll want to know about right now.

Whether you're just getting into biohacking, or you're a veteran biohacker, or you haven't even heard the term before, *The Spark Factor* can help you get the results you seek. It can help you heal chronic conditions or push the envelope of human achievement. It will be exciting to see what kind of impact this book has on the biohacking world and beyond. I wholeheartedly recommend this book as a must read for women seeking to live at their full potential. Dr. Molly Maloof is on her way to becoming the matriarch of biohacking!

—*Dave Asprey*

# Introduction

There is a spark of life inside each of your cells that powers your body with electricity. Some call it chi, or prana, or life force. It's a concept that exists in every culture and mythology because it is universal, but it's not a myth. All life arises from this spark.

But for many of us—and especially for women—the demands of life have begun to dim that spark. We feel crushed by chronic, unrelenting stress. We live in an environment polluted by environmental toxins. We eat processed food that increases inflammation, interferes with hormone balance, destabilizes blood sugar, and disrupts our microbiome health. Life is so convenient that we don't need to get physically active. Many of us live sedentary lives, sitting at desks all day and in front of televisions or computers all night, and pay for it with disrupted circadian rhythms that interfere with sleep quality. We communicate digitally and don't spend as much time face-to-face, in person, with the reassuring and supportive influence of eye contact and physical touch.

Life as we know it moves by in a flash and feels lonely, and all of this contributes to a dimming of the spark that energizes our lives. This isn't just a metaphorical dimming. It is a measurable reduction in the energy output from our cells. Without that spark, we can't live as long or as well. This quelling of energy production at the cellular level threatens to reduce the bright spark that should animate us all.

But what if I told you it was possible to reignite your spark? You could have the energy to go for your dreams. You could have all the energy you need, during whatever life stage you are currently in, and you could extend and expand the best years of your life, remaining vibrant and sharp as you age. You could maximize your quality of life, increase your happiness, and reduce your risk of developing chronic disease. Harnessing your spark is the key to reaching your physical, mental, and spiritual potential, and *biohacking*—intentionally manipulating your biology to optimize your health—is a method for doing just that.

Welcome to *The Spark Factor*. My career has spanned being a concierge doctor, Stanford lecturer, entrepreneur, and professional biohacker. I have provided personalized medicine services to high-performing technology executives, billionaire investors, Silicon Valley entrepreneurs, and Academy Award–winning actors. These are people who are passionate about experimenting with how to hack lifespan (how long you live) and healthspan (how long you remain healthy and functional) using cutting-edge technology and research. Nobody is more invested, literally, in hacking human healthspan and lifespan than the tech entrepreneurs in Silicon Valley, and many of them call on me to help them maximize their energy potential so they can stay as brilliant as possible for as long as possible.

These people have ambitious longevity goals. They want to live to a hundred and beyond without losing their mental sharpness or their physical fitness, and many of them are involved with companies that are investigating how to make that scenario a reality—companies I often advise, so I am on the ground floor of new technology and innovations. My patients tend to have a high level of privilege that affords them access to interventions unavailable in conventional medicine. But the exciting news is, these barriers to entry are starting to crumble.

Biohacking is going mainstream as more people begin to embrace the idea that you can manipulate your own health and performance.

Technology platforms are turning many of the personalized solutions I have offered my patients into scalable products and services. For example, personalized supplements, personalized probiotics, nutrigenomics, continuous glucose monitoring, and continuous heart rate variability monitoring—all of which were niche services ten years ago—are now available as consumer products. And they are becoming increasingly affordable, too, as more people discover the benefits of tracking their own biology to achieve their health, wellness, and performance goals.

And while biohacking is sometimes rooted in the latest technology, it can also be low-tech and tech-free, depending on what you want to impact and how far you want to take it. Even the simplest biohacks can transform your health, brighten your spark, charge your cellular batteries, and change your life for the better. Who wouldn't want in?

## How I Became a Biohacker

In some ways, I think I always had the personality for biohacking. I grew up in Peoria, Illinois, a precocious child, extremely headstrong and at the same time a good Christian girl. I was both well-behaved and rebellious, always trying to find creative solutions around anything in my way. I was an overachiever, but at least once a year, I would be sent to the principal's office for some infraction. In my defense, I didn't know I was breaking the rules. I remember once writing my name on the playground and a bunch of other kids did the same after me. Only when I was scolded for this did I learn the word *graffiti*. I think I was literally trying to leave my mark and didn't see what was so bad about that.

I was generally a happy kid, but I dealt with a lot of health problems. I suffered from multiple infections—ear infections, strep throat, pneumonia, and tonsillitis. Some of my earliest memories are of being in the hospital, something that I think contributed to my affinity for hospitals and my interest in practicing medicine.

Then, when I was about ten, my family experienced multiple tragedies in a short period of time. I was jolted out of childhood. I felt as if I became an adult overnight. I stopped playing with toys and started building my first mini business, sewing American Girl doll clothes and selling them at school. (Of course, this resulted in more visits to the principal's office.) I wanted to be self-sufficient, even at that young age.

This was also around the time I was assigned a book report on what I wanted to be when I grew up. I took this *very seriously*. I talked it over with my mom. I told her I was thinking about becoming a doctor but that I didn't know any girl doctors. She said, "You know, the doctor who delivered you and your sisters is a woman." Once I realized I could be a doctor too, I committed to this path, and I found a lot of comfort in knowing I had found my purpose. I started reading books written by doctors. Michael Crichton was a favorite. I also got into Russian literature because Chekhov was a doctor and both Tolstoy and Solzhenitsyn wrote about doctors.

By age eleven, I started going through puberty and my hormones were all over the place. My pre-teen years were awkward and confusing. I remember thinking, "Someday I'm going to figure out why all these things are happening to me, and I'm going to find a way to fix them."

At age thirteen, I found the book *Becoming a Physician* at the bookstore and got started on outlining my path. The next year I got to high school, and I threw myself into creating the kind of academic résumé I thought a future doctor would require. Because of my high drive and intense focus, I sacrificed my sleep to study. I became interested in supplements, trying to hack my biology before the word *biohacking* existed.

Once I got to college, I continued to design my life around what I thought would help me become a doctor. I joined all the relevant clubs.

I volunteered in hospitals, did research, worked in multiple libraries, and focused on learning how to learn.

That was probably the most influential thing I did—once I learned how to learn, I was able to take any syllabus and read any book and teach myself anything. That's when the whole world changed for me, academically and intellectually. Learning how to learn is learning how to solve your own problems by deconstructing them so you can customize solutions. I would watch recorded lectures and hardly ever go to class (my problems with focus made it hard for me to pay attention in large auditoriums), but my grades were high. You could say I hacked my undergrad degree.

Little did I know that in doing this, I was laying a foundation for my future as a biohacker, because that is exactly what biohacking is all about: solving your own body problems and figuring out how to reach your own health goals. It can save you time, and the time of any experts you may decide to consult, if you already know what's going on and what you want to fix. It's like a cheat code, so you don't have to start at square one every time you want somebody else's medical opinion.

When at last I made it to medical school, Dr. Ali, the doctor who delivered me and was my first inspiration to become a doctor, taught me how to perform a C-section during my OB-GYN rotation. It was an incredible moment, coming full circle like that. But medical school was grueling, as anybody who has gone through it knows. Halfway through med school, I was miserable and really struggling. I burned out.

In med school, there was no time for recovery. I started to get average grades, and I wasn't happy; I had terrible test anxiety. I didn't feel like myself, so I went to a psychologist and asked him if I had anxiety or depression. I wanted to understand what was wrong with me.

He saw exactly what was going on. Calmly he said, "You're fine, you're just a stressed-out medical student who's not taking care of herself." I realized *I* was the cause of my poor performance. I wasn't paying attention to my health, and so my energy capacity wasn't sufficient for the demands I was putting on myself. I needed to recharge my batteries.

I was thrilled to know that this was a problem I could do something about. I decided to research everything I could about how to live an evidence-based healthy life. Where was I draining my energy, and how could I replenish it? It didn't take long for me to figure out that lack of exercise, too much coffee, poor food choices, and not enough sleep were undoing me. I also wasn't spending nearly enough time with family or friends. I wasn't getting replenished with human connection. All of these habits accumulated to create a dysfunctional state of insufficient energy capacity.

I began to make changes. I started sleeping normal hours, eating consistently, doing yoga, meditating, and spending more time with my family. (As we'll soon discuss, these are all biohacks that can help recharge your energy at the cellular level.) As I began to alter my lifestyle, I could feel myself changing. I was happier, and my grades went up, too. After roughly six months of consistently practicing my new self-care regimen, I was transformed. I'd taken my first board exam the year before and my score was average, but when I took my second board exam, I was in the ninety-ninth percentile.

My classmates couldn't believe it and wanted to know what I did to raise my score so dramatically. "I changed my lifestyle," I told them. Those test results were a crystal-clear, objective measure of the changes I'd been making, and I couldn't believe nobody was teaching this to students. (I ended up designing a course for this exact purpose, when I was still a medical student, that became part of the school's curriculum, and for three years taught a similar course at Stanford designed to help students optimize their performance through lifestyle changes.)

As I reflected back on how far I'd come between those two board exams, I realized that I'd been stressed and anxious for pretty much my entire life. As soon as I started doing the right things for my health, as soon as I started increasing my energy capacity rather than draining it, I was able to take back control of my mind and body and flourish like never before. The equation is simple: greater energy = greater performance.

## Becoming a Biohacker

Once I finally became a doctor and began my residency, I found myself frustrated by the limits of the conventional healthcare system, which felt more focused on triaging illness than making people healthy. Why would I want to get entrenched in a system that profits from illness rather than teaching people how to create health? Why would I want to work within a system that doesn't pay for patients to get lab tests when they're healthy but is happy to pay for them when they're already sick? I began to doubt my path. I was very inspired by Dr. Andrew Weil so I researched his career path and realized he left his residency and went on to found the Institute of Integrative Medicine. After much deliberation, I took a leap of faith, completed my intern year of my residency, got my medical license, and started my own practice dedicated to optimizing health.

When I first got into biohacking, a colleague warned me, "Molly, you don't want to be known as a biohacker because that means you're trying to bypass the healthcare system instead of going through the system and working with it." But that's exactly what I wanted to do! I made a deliberate decision to step outside of the system and its focus on treating diseases, and step into the realm of upgrading human potential.

This is where the promise of true health lies. For example, I measure labs early and often on all my clients. By the time a serious problem shows up on lab tests and is diagnosable, it's likely been there for a while, slowly developing over years. I like to get ahead of these problems by knowing what's going on so I can predict and prevent disease.

Would you want to fly on an airplane that gets repaired only when it's already in the air? No, you would want the airplane to have sensors and be thoroughly checked *before* it goes out for a flight. The human body is like that airplane, and biohacking is about applying those sensors and doing that maintenance and knowing how that airplane works so you can avoid a crash. That data is feedback that can detect if your "plane" is going to go down in five years, rather than in five days or five minutes, because by then it may be too late.

Biohacking can unlock your understanding that you have been gifted with a power source that originates within your cells. As a woman, you have a uniquely creative energetic power (whether you use it to have children, start a company, grace the world with your art, or perform other meaningful work), and biohacking is a way to expand that creative energy potential so you can fulfill your destiny and purpose in this life, whatever that may be.

There are many complexities, difficulties, and joys inherent to being a woman, and another purpose for this book is to help you discover, contend with, and optimize life as a woman in the twenty-first century. That means I'll be talking about birth control and fertility, sex and love, food and exercise, and stress as they apply to a woman's unique biology. I'll also show you how biohacking—as interesting and complex as it is already—is even more interesting and complex for women, because of the cyclical nature of our lives.

As you embark upon this journey, I want to emphasize that the goal is steady gradual improvement, not perfection. My hope for you is that you can learn ways to optimize your biology so you can perform at your job or heal from illness or injury or take care of your family or just feel amazing as you live the life you've chosen to live. To do any of these things, you need ample energy. The goal is to help get your spark back so you can spend the rest of your life empowered, alive, mobile, and resilient.

NOTE: Throughout this book I will refer to various technologies, supplements, apps, lab tests, and more. I've created a website that offers guidance on all of my favorite brands and biohacking resources: https://drmolly.co/thesparkfactor/.

PART I

# THE HUMAN ENERGY CRISIS

# CHAPTER I

# Energy Powers Life

While risk reduction and health maintenance are noble, it is time to move the focus and efforts toward positive health potential through improved physical, mental, and social capabilities.

— Craig Becker and William Mcpeck[1]

Energy. It starts at the very beginning, when sperm meets egg. Scientists have captured on camera a fluorescent green zinc spark that flashes when an egg is fertilized.[2] Shortly after fertilization, the egg's mitochondria begin to do the work of powering embryo development. Mitochondria are cellular organelles that act as the powerhouses of the cell. They store electrical charge like batteries. Keeping our spark bright throughout our lives is a function of how well our mitochondria are able to create, store, and use energy. Without enough energy, the body can't do the work it needs to do. It can't fuel life. The strength of your spark and your capacity for energy creation determine how healthy you are.

You may already have a sense about the general state of your spark. Do you feel energetic when you wake up in the morning? Throughout the day? Or do you run out of energy before the day is over? Do you live with pain? That can be a sign of energy deficiency. Do you glow with health? That is a sign of good energy capacity. Is your energy capacity sufficient for what your life, and the world, demands of you? Most of the women I treat would answer no.

In fact, one of the leading complaints in doctors' offices today is fatigue. I've certainly noticed this shift, and so have my colleagues. Many people now consider it normal to be tired all the time, to be susceptible to viruses, and to have mood issues and exaggerated stress reactions, but none of this is normal. In my sickest patients with fatigue, I almost always see a similar pattern: a lifestyle that contradicts the principles of health and contributes to energy deficiency and immune system dysfunction. They get hit with a big stressful event, catch a nasty infection, and don't recover to their previous energy level. They stay at a suboptimal level of health.

When you don't have enough energy, you can feel it. Your brain can't function optimally, your body can't operate efficiently, and your life can feel more difficult, strenuous, and unsatisfying. If you aren't sick yet, over time, sustained insufficient energy production will almost certainly result in illness. Energy is the primary underlying factor in both longevity (length of life) and healthspan (length of health). If you want to live long and enjoy your life right now and right up to the end, expanding your energy capacity to brighten your spark is where to put your focus.

## Length of Life vs. Length of Health

Your healthspan is the portion of your life that you live without disease or disability, during which you remain vital, mobile, engaged, and cognitively sharp, and it is a function of energy production. The more energy you produce in your cells, the better your body will function and the longer you will remain healthy. People tend to think about and focus on lifespan, using drugs and surgery to prop up health while enduring a process of slow breakdown and decay. But if you lengthen your healthspan, you'll get more years of active, energized, and disease-free life. Isn't that what we all really want?

When we look at the health profiles of the longest-lived humans (the supercentenarians who live past 110), we see clearly that they eventually develop the same chronic diseases most people get. The critical difference between these people and the general population is that those who live the longest become sick only in the last few years of their lives—and sometimes only in the last few months or weeks. They have a long healthspan.

By contrast, chronic disease decline is typically long and slow, causing decades of disability and pain before the end. That's how most people go, so it may seem inevitable, but the truth is that in most cases, whether or not you will spend the last few decades of your life in decline is *not* predetermined. In fact, it is mostly self-determined. How you live now—how you build and maintain your energy capacity—will determine how you live later.

There is a long-standing belief that longevity is inherited, but according to the most recent research, only about 10 to 20 percent of the factors that influence your lifespan have a genetic basis.[3] Lifespan in the U.S. has increased by about 60 percent since 1900, due in part to the reduction in infectious disease–related deaths as a result of public health interventions like sewage and wastewater treatment, food safety, vaccines, antibiotics, and changing cultural views of personal hygiene.[4] But since 2014, when the average life expectancy in the U.S. was 78.9 years of age, lifespan has been trending downward again.[5] According to the CDC,[6] life expectancy in the U.S. in 2020 was 77.3 years of age (averaging men and women—women's lifespan is always a bit higher). Life expectancy dropped by another 1.5 years in 2020 due to the COVID-19 pandemic, but that just sped up what was happening already. The U.S. is shockingly low on the list of developed countries when it comes to lifespan. (Japan is the highest.)

If you look at the actual causes of death over the last decade, you can see that modifiable behavioral risk factors (e.g., poor diet, physical inactivity, smoking, drinking, excess stress, social disconnection, etc.) underlie most of the chronic diseases that are killing us. Take the number one cause of death, heart disease, which kills more women and men than any other disease and costs about $1 billion every day in medical costs and productivity losses.[7] Heart disease often strikes in middle age—a surprising number of people have heart attacks between the ages of thirty-five and sixty-four—but according to the American Heart Association, 80 percent of cardiovascular disease, including heart disease and stroke, is preventable.[8] Cancer, another common cause of death, may also be at least 50 percent preventable[9] through strategies like quitting smoking, eating a more nutritious diet, drinking less alcohol, getting vaccinated against viruses like hepatitis and the human papillomavirus (HPV), and taking measures to protect against skin cancer.

Then there is diabetes, which is startlingly common in the U.S. More than 10 percent of Americans have diabetes, one in three has prediabetes, and rates are rising fastest among young people.[10] But only 10 to 15 percent of type 2 diabetes risk is genetic, which means that the development of this disease is highly influenced by lifestyle, socioeconomic, and environmental factors. Tragically, 84 percent of people who have prediabetes aren't aware of it, and 21 percent of people with diabetes are undiagnosed.[11]

Most twenty-first-century humans have lifestyles and environments that create the conditions for mitochondrial dysfunction. This impairs metabolism, leads to insufficient energy capacity, sets off inflammatory alarm signals, ages us prematurely—and results in the development of chronic disease. Because mitochondria—organelles inside of our cells—produce energy, the number and health of our mitochondria determine our energy capacity. That is why I call the mitochondria our "batteries." Compromise your battery capacity and you compromise your health, because your body has less energy to devote to keeping you well.

It is true that there will always be a percentage of the population who, for some reason, become sick despite what their genetics and lifestyle should predict. But it's also true that most people can prevent or delay the onset of chronic metabolic disease by maximizing energy capacity and minimizing energy drain.

Since most people today are living with suboptimal energy production, it's not surprising that, according to the National Center for Chronic Disease Prevention and Health Promotion, 60 percent of Americans already have at least one chronic disease.[12] I'm not trying to live to 150 like many Silicon Valley longevity seekers. What I care about is maintaining my *quality* of life for as long as I possibly can. At some point, our lives will end, but the end of a functional body and a functional brain does not have to precede the end of life—at least, not by as much as we tend to think.

If you start optimizing your energy capacity when you're still healthy (or even just fairly healthy or somewhat healthy), you could significantly delay the onset of disease and disability. You can square off the healthspan curve, ensuring a better quality of life for longer. If you are lucky, you may end up as one of those supercentenarians who celebrate their 110th birthday in good health.

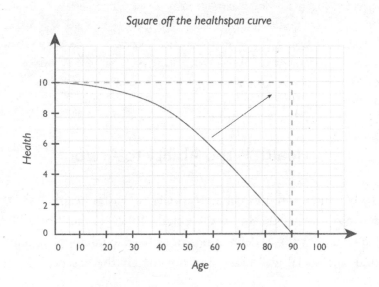

*Square off the healthspan curve*

Increasing healthspan to the maximum possible requires that you stop doing things that compromise energy capacity and start doing things that increase energy capacity. It's really that straightforward. If you want to build health, live longer, and lengthen your healthspan, the goal is to build your energy capacity by optimizing your mitochondrial function. Create more and bigger batteries with more capacity to store energy, keep them charged, and use them wisely. That's how you get your spark back. And that, at its crux, is the foundation of health.

## ANCIENT GENETICS IN MODERN BODIES

Humans have always had to contend with stressors, but the stress we face today is different from the stress faced by our ancestors. We live in an artificial (electrically powered, indoor) and profoundly polluted environment, out of sync with the natural rhythms of the sun and seasons. We live in a culture that emphasizes pleasure and convenience while also demanding extreme productivity and perfection. We exist often in isolation from extended family, communicating with friends and family through screens, and hunched over devices with little to no awareness of the outside world. We have developed a modernized human existence that directly contradicts our genetic adaptations. We are not made to be sedentary, to overeat, to never fast, to experience chronic, unrelenting stress, to have sunlight-mimicking screens in our faces at night, to resist feeling our emotions, or to live alone with no meaningful tribe. It's a genetic mismatch that is out of alignment with nature and directly compromises energy production, reducing quality and length of life.

## Health Is the Ability to Adapt

To truly understand how energy capacity underlies health, let's take a closer look at what "health" really entails. In 1948, the World Health Organization (WHO) defined health as "a state of complete physical, mental, and social well-being and not merely the absence of disease or infirmity."[13] That's a high bar, and a pretty unrealistic one. Humans tend to catch viruses, break parts of themselves, and generally experience wear and tear with age, especially if they live life vigorously. Who would you say is healthier: the person who sits in a chair all day eating salad and taking no risks, or the person who climbs mountains, dives into oceans, and travels the world, and because of all that, has suffered from stress fractures, ruptured tendons, and the occasional rogue virus? Part of understanding what health is, is to think about what health is to *you*. How do *you* want to use your energy? What do *you* want to get out of your life? Do you value safety or adventure? A contemplative life or a dangerous one?

Taking this personalization into account, I think the best, most accurate description of health I've seen comes from Machteld Huber's 2011 definition[14] of health as "the ability to adapt and self-manage in the face of social, physical, and emotional challenges." That is how I define health—the ability to adapt to adversity. Life is constantly hitting us with challenges, and how we react and adapt to those challenges is the real marker of health. Our health is tested by our capacity to handle major stressors and be resourced emotionally, physically, spiritually, and socially to bounce back and continue to thrive.

Unfortunately, too many women are already in the process of mental and physical breakdown. They aren't adapting. If you have a chronic disease, you aren't adapting. If you're tired all the time, you aren't adapting. If you can't stop overeating or undersleeping, overworking or underperforming, overstressing or underexercising, isolating or obsessing over social media, running on caffeine and fumes or self-medicating with alcohol or other substances, you aren't adapting.

Why don't we know how to adapt to adversity? That's the four-trillion-dollar question (because that's the amount of money people spent on healthcare in 2020[15]). People—especially women—are tired, worried, burned out, and stressed. We push ourselves to overachieve, agonize over the future, and feel paralyzed by a fear of failure (or a fear of success). Many of my female friends and followers describe dealing with the insidious effects of trauma, clinical depression, debilitating anxiety, and an inner battle about the basic worth of and ownership over their own bodies. Something is obviously wrong, but we see few mainstream solutions other than vague general advice like "Lose some weight" or "Get more sleep" or "Try not to be so stressed." And these issues are affecting younger populations than ever before. According to the American Psychological Association,[16] millennials and Gen Z report the most stress of any age group. It used to be that the youngest adults had the brightest spark. That has been compromised by the human energy crisis.

But there is hope. Even if your doctor isn't telling you what to do about your undiagnosable, vague, life-compromising symptoms of energy depletion, there is plenty you can do on your own. You can start slowly and gradually build your energy capacity back up again. You can make more batteries, keep them charged, and use them in a way that increases their capacity rather than draining it. This is how you create a more resilient body that *can* adapt and manage in the face of adversity. This is how you turn up your spark.

## Assessing Your Spark

If you were a video game character, what would your energy level look like right now? Are your levels topped off, or are you on the last of your lives? Imagine you encounter an opponent, and you lose all your energy. If you have multiple lives, you might live to fight another day, with a fresh tank, as you keep playing and achieving greater energy levels with greater skills mastered. But if you don't build up your energy levels, you're not going to get to play the game for very long.

Understanding this concept is the key to unlocking the techniques in this book. If you think about your energy capacity, as measured by your mitochondrial health, in those terms, it can be easy to conceptualize what lowers your energy level and what fills you up. You have to build your health every day, like a muscle, to keep increasing your energy capacity, and you build it by way of the choices you make. The more capacity you build, the more dividends you reap and the better you can adapt to stressors.

## AVOIDING THE "HEALTHCARE" SYSTEM

One of the best reasons to be healthy might simply be to avoid having to use the "healthcare" system. But let's call it what it is: a sickness billing-industrial complex. Today's medical system is designed to code for disease, disability, and death, and charge you for services to manage your care rather than reverse chronic illness. Healthcare costs a lot of money, and it doesn't give you or your doctor autonomy. Once doctors are in practice, they become subcontractors of insurance companies, whether they like it or not. They aren't incentivized to practice in a way that promotes health and flourishing. The system doesn't educate them on nutrition or lifestyle medicine, so most doctors today are not equipped to approach health in this way, anyway.

What's more, the U.S. healthcare system is based on a militaristic, bureaucratic structure that requires physicians to sacrifice an enormous amount of their lives and their own health to care for others. I say this from a perspective of personal experience because I was once a part of this system. Burnout is pervasive because most physicians are operating at an unhealthy capacity due to the great burden of disease in the populations they treat. Doctors have some of the highest rates of suicide of all professions.[17] Their energy drain exceeds their energy capacity, and they break down.

It is absolutely crazy that we let our economy (18 percent of our GDP) depend on the sickness of our society. Do you really want to rely on overworked doctors operating in an antiquated and ineffective system? When you really need them, you will really need them, but with biohacking and a lifestyle that promotes energy capacity and resilience, you can significantly influence whether you'll ever have to rely on the healthcare system for more than crisis intervention.

Before I started taking my health seriously, I was drinking way too much caffeine, I didn't sleep well, and I never exercised. I was lazy with my nutrition—I would eat cereal as a meal (multiple times a day). I had no stress management practice and I had tons of anxiety. I wasn't building up my energy levels with sleep, exercise, and good food. I was draining my energy levels. After I started cutting back to a cup of coffee a day, sleeping regularly, doing yoga daily, eating a more plant-focused diet with balanced nutrition, and meditating regularly, I was able to do more work with less effort.

Understanding how to do that requires knowing where you are, then setting goals for where you want to be. You can start by frankly assessing your energy levels right now. Here are some signs that you have insufficient energy capacity:

- **RUNNING OUT OF ENERGY BEFORE THE DAY IS OVER.** Do you feel like you need a nap (or a double espresso) halfway through the day? If you can't make it to bedtime without feeling like you're dragging, that's an obvious sign of drained batteries.

- **GROGGY MORNINGS.** How do you feel when you wake up in the morning? A lot of people can't get out of bed without an alarm. Waking up naturally and feeling good in the morning is a sign of high energy and good health.

- **POOR SLEEP.** Do you sleep peacefully throughout the night or do you wake up frequently? Sleeping soundly through the night and feeling refreshed in the morning is a marker of energy capacity and an important way to charge your cellular batteries.

- **GENERALLY UNSTABLE MOOD.** If you often feel erratic, have mood swings, or feel anxiety or depression, these are consequences of poor health or health problems. Low energy capacity has negative effects on the brain. Your brain uses more energy than any other organ in the body, so when your energy system fails, so will your brain.

- INABILITY TO FOCUS. If you are struggling with focusing on work and finding it hard to concentrate, this is another sign of energy deficiency. Brain fog and the inability to manage a complex life are signs that the brain isn't getting a steady stream of energy.

- NEEDING TO EAT ALL THE TIME. This could be a sign of stress, blood sugar regulation problems, or a high-carb, low-nutrient diet contributing to metabolic inflexibility, or difficulty switching from burning carbs to burning fat. Over time, this leads to reduced energy capacity. Overeating is one of the quickest ways to compromise mitochondrial health.

- POOR RELATIONSHIP QUALITY. This one may not seem directly related to health, but if you don't have at least several deep relationships with other people, it will be very difficult to be truly healthy. Healthy, supportive relationships greatly reduce stress and improve quality of life. Not having these can seriously compromise energy capacity.

- LOW STAMINA, ENDURANCE, AND STRENGTH. If you have issues with stamina, endurance, and strength, those are direct reflections of a lack of sufficient energy. With a lot of energy capacity, you'll have an easier time with exercise, even when you're just getting started. If you struggle with a few flights of stairs, your mitochondria need attention.

- FLEXIBILITY AND BONE STRENGTH. Weak bones and stiff joints are a sign of declining energy that is compromising your structure.

- DULL SENSES. Your senses are related to nerve function. Good vision, hearing, sense of taste and smell, and sensitivity to touch are reflective of strong electrical "wiring." Dull senses mean the wiring isn't working.

- DULL SKIN. When you look at somebody who's really vibrant and healthy, they look like they emit light (even as they age). This is called skin autofluorescence. Compare that to somebody who looks sallow or who has poor skin quality, whether that's cystic acne, excessive wrinkles, or dullness. These are signs that there is some form of hormone dysfunction (often due to insulin resistance). People who suffer from diabetes and have impaired mitochondrial function have skin that emits less light than healthy people's.[18]

- VISCERAL FAT. While many look to the number on the scale as a marker of health, what matters more is the type of fat you have. A little bit of excess weight isn't going to harm you, but if you have visceral fat (the fat that gets packed around your organs)—even if you are slender— then that is a marker of poor health. This is best measured by a DEXA scan or MRI, but it's also indicative of visceral fat if you are a woman and your waist size is greater than thirty-five inches (or greater than forty inches for a man).

- BRITTLE HAIR OR NAILS. These are external markers of health, like leaves on a tree or a plant. Droopy, dead, or shedding leaves (out of season) on a tree are signs that the tree isn't healthy, and stress-related hair loss or dry, brittle, or prematurely gray hair[19] (defined as having gray hair before the age of twenty in Europeans, before twenty-five in Asians, and before thirty in Africans) can be a sign of mitochondrial dysfunction.

If you checked multiple boxes on this list, you are probably suffering from insufficient energy capacity, and it's most likely due to your lifestyle. There are four basic factors that reduce energy capacity and four basic factors that increase it. Think about how you are doing in each of these areas:

**REDUCES ENERGY CAPACITY**

1. *Inactivity*
2. *Overeating and poor nutrition causing chronic inflammation*
3. *Too much stress*
4. *Social disconnection*

**INCREASES ENERGY CAPACITY**

1. *Exercise and recovery, to build cellular batteries*
2. *Eating the right foods in the right amounts at the right times, to charge cellular batteries*
3. *Effective stress management with sufficient sleep, meditation, and nature exposure, to properly use cellular batteries*
4. *Human touch and connection, to plug in and thrive*

Throughout this book, I'll share biohacking strategies to help you overcome the challenges on the first list and embrace the habits on the second list, so you can maximize your energy production to increase your healthspan.

## Preparing to Pursue Health

Energy is the foundation. Biohacking is the means. Health will be the result. It's not complicated, but it requires a commitment to create health within yourself.

Pursuing health may sound like something everyone would want to do, but when it comes to making actual lifestyle changes, the reality can be more difficult than the concept. You know you should exercise and eat more vegetables, but what if you just don't have the energy to do what it takes to create energy? Or what if you simply lack the material or emotional resources required to thrive?

You can only start where you are and work to the best of your ability to take steps in the right direction. But that's all you need to do. You can invest a lot of time or a little. You can spend a lot of money or none. You can have big goals or small goals. It's your path. Whatever you want to do or can do, this book can help you do it *your* way. Biohacking is ultimately personal. It's about learning to listen to your own internal wisdom, whether you do that with fancy tech or just by getting quiet with yourself and paying attention.

The energetic changes I've experienced by biohacking my health have been incredible, inside and out. I have more energy, better focus, better digestion, and a sharper mind than I've ever had before (not to mention, my hair is thicker, my nails are stronger, and my skin is clearer—these are external markers of health). But to really inspire you to embark upon this journey with me, let's look at some compelling reasons why making an effort (and I'm not going to pretend it's not an effort) to pursue health is worthwhile. These are three bigger-picture advantages to actively pursuing health that you may not have thought much about before:

- **SURVIVAL/GAINING EVOLUTIONARY FITNESS.** Simply put, if you're healthy, you will be better able to run away if you need to, less likely to fall, and more able to lift heavy things (you never know when that might be a matter of life and death), fight off a threat, or think your way out of a bad situation. You'll also have a more discerning immune system to fight off viruses, bacteria, and cancer cells that might try to take you down. Your heart, lungs, blood vessels, liver, kidneys, and pancreas will be stronger, so you'll be less likely to get heart disease, lung disease, atherosclerosis, liver and kidney disease, and diabetes. You'll have strong joints and dense bones, so you'll be less likely to have a life-threatening accident, break a hip, or be crippled by arthritis. If you desire a family, your reproductive health is likely to be stronger. You'll also be in a much better position to compete for the life you want in a world that still prioritizes the needs of men.

- **HAVING OPTIONS, CHOICES, FREEDOM, AND THE CAPACITY AND INNER RE-SOURCES TO DO MEANINGFUL WORK.** Health gives you more possibilities and options. Energy helps you do more of what you want with your life, and that is what can give your life meaning. That could look like going to college, or building a company, or supporting others in your community. Whatever it is that is meaningful to you, energy capacity and the health it creates can be just what you need to commit yourself to your own life, your relationships, and your mission.

- **HAVING A BETTER QUALITY OF LIFE.** Health means greater productivity, better efficiency, and less fatigue, so whatever you are doing, you can feel better and enjoy yourself more while you're doing it. You'll have increased focus and improved executive function, be in a better mood, sleep more peacefully at night, have inner calm and confidence in your abilities, live free of chronic pain, and maintain your autonomy as you age, since you will be less likely to be physically dependent on others.

Health is a means to an end that goes beyond just surviving. It's the fuel for achieving your goals, actualizing your purpose, and achieving your potential. You can learn how to prepare your body for worst-case scenarios and monitor your body so that you can intervene before minor issues became serious problems. You can feel amazing rather than just okay. You can feel awake to your life rather than foggy and tired. And you can start right now.

# CHAPTER 2

# Mitochondria

## YOUR CELLULAR BATTERIES

Your 40 trillion cells contain at least a quadrillion mitochondria, with a combined convoluted surface area of about 14,000 square metres; about four football fields. Their job is to pump protons, and together they pump more than $10^{21}$ of them—nearly as many as there are stars in the known universe—every second.

—Nick Lane

We are collectively experiencing a human energy crisis, and, at its root, the fatigue that plagues so many of us is a result of mitochondrial dysfunction. When the powerhouses of the cell stop operating properly, energy deficiency follows, and energy deficiency precedes all chronic disease, so in many ways, biohacking health really comes down to biohacking mitochondria.

We have a bidirectional relationship with these tiny energy producers: they influence everything about our experience of life, and they are influenced by everything we do. Fortunately for us, their sensitivity to their environment means that it's relatively straightforward to hack our mitochondria, to start increasing energy and start improving health almost immediately.

## How Mitochondria Generate Power

There is a widely accepted theory that mitochondria evolved from bacterial life-forms that, over the course of evolution, were absorbed by host cells to help them better harvest energy from their environment. Through this symbiotic relationship, the extra energy these bacteria created for the host organism enabled the evolution of higher and more complex forms of life. Mitochondria may have played an instrumental role in human evolution. What was once a symbiotic relationship between two separate organisms is now a mutually beneficial fusion of two into one.

But mitochondria are not human. They are their own organisms. They have their own DNA. We are interdependent but separate. Considering you are serving as their host, you might want to understand a little more about these "tenants" who live in and on your body. Understanding how mitochondria work for you will help you understand how to optimize them, so let's dial in and take a closer look. (I promise I'll go easy on the really technical stuff, to keep you interested.)

Here's a basic question: where does energy originate from? If you take it all the way back, energy originally comes from the sun. Plants capture sunlight and store it as energy inside their cells. Animals eat plants, and the energy in those plants feeds the mitochondria in the animals, to make energy for them. Humans eat the animals and the plants, and our mitochondria harvest energy stored in the animals and plants we eat to make energy for us. Energy production itself is analogous to a solar-powered pump in a hydroelectric dam that pushes water slowly up the dam's reservoir. When energy is required, the dam opens, causing water to flow, and the turbine spins, producing energy.

In the case of mitochondria, that energy comes in the form of adenosine triphosphate, or ATP, the energy currency in our cells that is made, saved, and spent by our mitochondria. Mitochondria act as both batteries to store this energy and capacitors to deploy it. Our bodies spend energy produced by the cell doing work, whether that's at the cellular level (like cleaning the cell of waste) or beyond (like building our structure and using our muscles). Since we are made of cells, everything we do happens not just at the macro level that we see and perceive (cleaning the house, mowing the lawn, using our brains to work, having sex, running, talking . . . in other words, living) but at the cellular level, where the energy is being made. This is why, when mitochondria don't receive all the things they need to make energy, we notice. Lose energy at the cellular level, and you lose energy at the life level.

## LIGHTNING INSIDE YOUR CELLS

According to Douglas Wallace, PhD, the director of the Center for Mitochondrial and Epigenomic Medicine at the Children's Hospital of Philadelphia, mitochondria generate 90 percent of our cellular energy, and each mitochondrion holds 0.2 volts. Each of us has about $10^{17}$ mitochondria in our bodies, so that means you contain more potential energy than a lightning bolt![1]

While making energy is the primary function of the mitochondria, they do other things, too. They are involved in the oversight of critical biological processes across your entire system. For example, they direct much of your cellular housekeeping. They are in charge of apoptosis, or programmed cell death that eliminates potentially harmful cells, as well as mitophagy, which is the cleaning out of malfunctioning mitochondria that no longer carry a charge.

Mitochondria also influence how your energy is allocated through cellular signaling between phases of growth or breakdown of tissue such as muscle. Under times of threat, it helps produce more stress hormones so you can respond to emergencies better. Mitochondria will do everything in their power to protect your precious energy stores and commit them only to what is essential. When you feel safe and have enough essential nutrients, mitochondria help direct your resources to secondary functions like building muscle, digesting food, and procreating. This is why, when we are highly stressed, things like digestion, detoxification, fertility, and athletic performance can suffer, and we hold on to fat more stubbornly. It's harder to lose weight under stress because our bodies want to make sure we have enough energy available to get us through the perceived challenges.

## Mitochondria and Immunity

Mitochondria are instrumental in the body's immune response, and stress can compromise how effective mitochondria are at powering the immune system. If you aren't making enough energy due to chronic stress, your immune system won't get enough energy to work efficiently. Since the immune system serves to both detect and combat invaders like pathogens such as viruses and bacteria, it needs a lot of energy.

You can see how this plays out with chronic fatigue syndrome (CFS). In the summer of 2019, I was seeing a number of patients with CFS so I spent a good amount of time researching this condition (it's sometimes called myalgic encephalomyelitis). I discovered that almost all my patients had preexisting highly stressful lifestyles and either a major infection or series of previous infections, combined with an acute life stressor that completely broke down their health.

When these patients got hit with an infection, they couldn't respond to the invaders appropriately because they already had depleted energy. The bugs (e.g., viruses and other intracellular pathogens like Lyme, syphilis, rickettsia, etc.) were able to enter and hide inside the cells. Many viruses can hijack cellular machinery for their own purposes, which causes massive energy drain, inflammation, and fatigue. Some, like HIV, can even commandeer mitochondrial proteins, increasing their chances of replication inside the cell.[2] Once viruses enter the cell, they can replicate and kill the cell, releasing the viruses into the system.[3]

When this happens, we can often detect insufficient mitochondrial energy production. A 2020 study[4] found mitochondrial abnormalities in people with chronic fatigue syndrome. In an older study from 1991,[5] researchers took muscle biopsies of fifty patients between one and seventeen years of age who had been suffering from chronic fatigue syndrome after a viral infection and found obvious mitochondrial degeneration in the muscle fibers. Many people who have recovered from viruses continue to have prolonged chronic fatigue because of degenerated mitochondria.

After some research into all of this, I wondered why the mainstream health system doesn't pay more attention to chronic fatigue conditions and their link to viruses. In fact, in August 2019, I said to a friend, "We don't know enough about viruses, and we are way overdue for a plague." I had a feeling that if a viral plague were to happen, we would see massive amounts of chronic fatigue syndrome. When the pandemic hit in 2020, unfortunately I was not surprised by the emergence of chronic or "long-haul" COVID. The COVID-19 virus can enter and infect cells. This infection causes massive mitochondrial dysfunction, inflammation and oxidative stress that damages cells leading to downstream organ dysfunction, especially in the lungs. The way I see it, inflammation is like fire, oxidative stress is like smoke, and mitochondrial dysfunction is like the power getting cut.

This is why you see global manifestations of disease and debilitating fatigue across all body systems with long-haul COVID. The most mitochondrial-rich and most energy-demanding organs (the heart and brain) display the most obvious problems (e.g., heart palpitations, myocarditis, brain fog, tinnitus, and loss of smell). Muscle cells are also rich in mitochondria, which is why general fatigue and fatigue with exercise are so common in chronic fatigue syndrome and chronic COVID.

I'm often asked how to fix long-haul COVID or chronic fatigue syndrome. This is an active area of research right now and we are sure to learn more about it as more results come in, but for now, if you are currently suffering from some of the effects of chronic or long-haul

COVID, these are some of the interventions I recommend to help improve mitochondrial function after viral infection:

- LYMPHATIC DRAINAGE. You can work on lymphatic drainage on your own by sweating in a sauna, dry brushing, doing self-massage, foam rolling, walking, and doing yoga, or you can see a practitioner who specializes in lymphatic drainage massage. These practices help pump lymph fluid through the body, which helps with detoxification and immunity.

- BREATHING EXERCISES. Breathing practices are important for helping to heal the lungs and restore proper lung capacity following a respiratory infection. Respiratory muscle training involves using an incentive spirometer (a handheld resistance device to practice forced expiration, which you can get from your doctor). Cough exercises involve performing ten active coughs a day. Various breathwork practices can also help relieve stress while recovering from infection. See a few I like on page 199.

- ANTI-INFLAMMATORY DIET. COVID-19 involves massive inflammatory injury to the body, so it's important to eat an anti-inflammatory diet. Eat a lot of colorful vegetables, along with some fruit, legumes, fatty fish, grass-fed lean protein or wild game, spices, and nuts and seeds, and consume few or no refined grains and processed foods. It's also especially important to avoid any known food sensitivities. (For more on diet, see chapters 6 through 9.)

- OZONE THERAPY. In low concentrations, ozone can boost antioxidant systems and aid in clearing stubborn infections. This isn't something you can do on your own. To get this therapy, look for a reputable functional medicine doctor who uses ozone therapy regularly in their practice.

- **HBOT.** This stands for "hyperbaric oxygen therapy." Spending time at high pressure in an HBOT tank promotes healing, enhances mitochondrial function, and clears infections. This requires an appointment with a practitioner.

- **TOXIN AVOIDANCE.** One of the most important things you can do to optimize mitochondrial function is to avoid things that directly damage mitochondria including household mold exposure, alcohol, certain drugs (e.g. antibiotics, acetaminophen, cocaine, amphetamine, NSAIDs, and statins), heavy metals like mercury, pesticides, persistent organic pollutants (in unfiltered tap water), excessive EMF exposure, phthalates and parabens (in beauty products).

- **SUPPLEMENTS.** A variety of supplements can be used to help manage symptoms following infection. I recommend working with a functional medicine doctor to help you design your optimal regimen. Some supplements I recommend:

  **ANTI-INFLAMMATORIES.** Supplements like vitamin D (5,000 IU with K1 & K2), melatonin at night (start with 1 mg), and curcumin (500–1,000 mg) all have anti-inflammatory effects. I take 4 grams of pharmaceutical grade fish oil a day for the pro-resolving mediators they contain, which are potent anti-inflammatories that can't be recapitulated by anything else, but check with your doctor to see if you are a candidate for high-dose prescription omega-3s.

  **MITOCHONDRIAL FUNCTION ENHANCERS.** For fatigue, supplements that enhance mitochondrial function are magnesium (400 mg/day), acetyl-L-carnitine (2 g/day), and pyrroloquinoline quinone (aka PQQ at 20 mg), a B-complex, creatinine (3 to 5 g/day), and coenzyme Q10 (100 mg/day).

**ELECTROLYTES.** For orthostatic hypotension (when your blood pressure drops if you stand up too quickly, causing dizziness and sometimes fainting), sufficient electrolytes are important. Add a pinch of pink Himalayan sea salt to your water.

**LUNG SUPPORT.** N-acetylcysteine (NAC) (500–1,000 mg/day) to support restoration of the body's glutathione stores. Glutathione is the body's primary internally made antioxidant and the most abundant antioxidant in the lungs. I also recommend vitamin C (1 g/day) and mullein, to help improve lung function.

**FOR PREVENTING BLOOD CLOTS,** I recommend nattokinase (4,000 SPU) or serratiopeptidase enzymes (40,000 SPU/day). Omega-3s also help to thin the blood.

**FOR BRAIN HEALTH,** try lion's mane for benefits to neuroplasticity (3 g/day seems to be the best dose for optimizing brain function).

**FOR DETOXIFICATION,** try liposomal glutathione (500–1,000 mg/day) and binder formulas containing activated charcoal, bentonite clay, modified citrus pectin, and chlorella. Home-grown broccoli sprouts are also great because they contain sulfurophane. And, don't forget to filter the air and water in your home.

If you want more information on this subject, my favorite book on the topic is *Diagnosis and Treatment of Chronic Fatigue Syndrome and Myalgic Encephalitis: It's Mitochondria, Not Hypochondria* by Dr. Sarah Myhill.

## How Habits Impact Mitochondria

Mitochondria are your partners in health because they are responsive and reactive to your lifestyle. They grow, multiply, or die off in accordance with their environment, and there are three primary behaviors that most dramatically degrade mitochondrial function:

1. **INSUFFICIENT MOVEMENT.** *A body that doesn't exercise or is sedentary is sending signals to the mitochondria that it doesn't need more energy, so the mitochondria will decrease energy production, especially in the muscles and heart. When you live in a way that demands more energy, by moving and exercising more, your mitochondria will respond by making more energy to meet your demand.*

2. **OVERCONSUMPTION.** *When you overeat, especially high-sugar foods, your cells release a kind of exhaust (reactive oxygen species) that can damage mitochondria and the lining of blood vessels. Fuel the body can't use gets stored in fat cells, which contributes to obesity, which further increases inflammation and other conditions that damage the mitochondria.*

3. **CHRONIC STRESS WITHOUT RECOVERY.** *Stress contributes to mitochondrial allostatic load (the cumulative stress load within a cell), which often drives maladaptive behaviors like drinking, smoking, and overeating, all of which further contribute to mitochondrial dysfunction. Without recovery, mitochondria don't get a chance to repair and recharge.*

### A SUPPLEMENT STRATEGY

Throughout this book, and in many areas on my website, I recommend supplement use. This can start to feel overwhelming if you see multiple lists of supplements (from me and elsewhere). To help you narrow it down and decide what's most important, you need a supplement strategy, rather than taking a bunch of things without a plan.

I use supplements in two ways in my practice. First is a baseline set of supplements I prescribe to cover the most common deficiencies: pharmaceutical-grade omega-3s, vitamin D, magnesium, B-complex, and a minerals complex. These are useful for general daily health maintenance, because your mitochondria and metabolism need nutrients to run properly. These are also what I almost always see are needed based on laboratory testing. I use urine organic acids, blood tests, and hair mineral testing results to personalize patients' supplement regimens. Organic acids and hair minerals are particularly good for identifying vitamin, mineral, and phytonutrient status. Under high stress, it's not uncommon to see $B_6$, sodium, and potassium deficiencies, which can manifest in fatigue. Your cells are batteries that run on mineral gradients and the body uses up more minerals when it's under a lot of stress. I always get a ferritin level on men and women because it is a marker of iron storage and iron is the mineral that allows your red blood cells to carry oxygen, which mitochondria need for cellular respiration. If ferritin is low (<75 ng/mL) I have patients supplement with iron. If ferritin is high (>150 ng/mL) this can cause oxidative stress, and I recommend patients go give blood to lower their iron.

I like to test before I supplement, but if you don't want to or can't do these tests, you can safely take these basic supplements even without testing. Some women just take prenatal vitamins to cover most of their bases.

The second way I use supplements is to optimize different systems, and this is even more personalized. I always begin with gut health because if someone has gut dysfunction, they may not be absorbing nutrients and will often have problems with hormones, because a compromised gut can't fully clear excess hormones through the stool. Gut dysfunction can also compromise immunity, and people with this problem often have food intolerances or allergies. Gut healing can take time—usually three months to really start seeing results (I'll talk about how to do this specifically in chapter 8).

Next, I would look at optimizing recovery from stress, and optimizing sleep and circadian rhythms, for those who have sleep issues. If hormones are still an issue, those will need to be addressed with supplements or bioidentical hormone replacement (I'll talk about both of those in chapter 12). Detoxification from heavy metals or mold toxicity may be required in those exposed. Then there are supplements used to optimize for mitochondrial health and aging.

The key point here is that you don't just use all the supplements all at once. Focus on a particular area of improvement over three to six months before optimizing the next area. There are all sorts of things that can interact when you take a boatload of supplements, and the body needs time to let them work and do their magic.

People often don't understand the serious repercussions of a mitochondria-damaging lifestyle. According to mitochondrial researcher Dr. Douglas Wallace, pathology (disease) emerges when energy capacity declines past 50 percent, which is the threshold of insufficient energy availability.[6] But there are things you can do to keep energy capacity above 50 percent. These five life-extending health habits can make you 82 percent less likely to die from cardiovascular disease and 65 percent less likely to die from cancer, and could prolong life expectancy at age 50 by an extra 14 years for women and 12.2 years for men,[7] because of (essentially) how they either enhance or degrade mitochondria:

1. **NOT SMOKING.** *Smoking directly damages mitochondrial quality and function because inhaling concentrated pollution directly into your bloodstream causes an extreme inflammatory response and oxidative stress.*

2. **EATING A HEALTHY DIET.** *A nutrient-rich, diverse diet provides your mitochondria with the vitamins, minerals, and cofactors they need to produce energy, and a phytonutrient-rich (plant-rich) diet enables your body to better process and eliminate waste that could otherwise linger in the body and damage mitochondria.*

3. **EXERCISING.** *When you exercise regularly, you send signals to your muscles to create more mitochondria, to meet the increased energy demands, especially when your exercise changes frequently and challenges muscles (including the heart muscle) and the brain.*

4. **MAINTAINING A HEALTHY BODY WEIGHT.** *Obesity overloads and overwhelms the mitochondria with fuel (fat and glucose), causing them to malfunction, which leads to inflammation and oxidative stress that further damage mitochondria.*

5. **MINIMIZING ALCOHOL CONSUMPTION.** *Drinking too much alcohol damages the liver, which is one of the most mitochondria-dense organs. The liver is responsible for blood sugar homeostasis and*

*cellular detoxification. When your liver is impaired, these processes are impaired.*

## Tune Your Mitochondria with Hormesis

If you want to have more energy capacity to defend against stress, immune suppression, viral infection, fatigue syndromes, and chronic diseases—if you want to become stronger in mind and body with a long, healthy life and extended healthspan—then you can choose, by the way you live, to actively defend your mitochondria and optimize your energetic capacity.

To do this you need to change the signals you are sending to your mitochondria. That means (1) doing things that challenge the mitochondria to increase energy production, and (2) allowing sufficient recovery time during which mitochondria can respond. This is a two-step process that is the basis for a mitochondria-enhancing practice called hormesis.

Hormesis refers to the positive effect of stressors. Yes, stress can be good. Specifically, hormesis means that small amounts of stress can generate a positive biological response. When dosed properly, stress is beneficial because it sends signals to your mitochondria that they need to step up energy production to meet what might be an ongoing demand. The mitochondria comply, and you get more energy and greater capacity to handle stress, which translates to greater resilience.

A good example of how hormesis works is weight lifting. When you lift heavy weights, you create microtears, or small injuries, in your mitochondria-dense muscles. In small doses, injuries can be beneficial, as long as they're followed by sufficient recovery time. The mitochondria get the signal that you are using your muscles, so they produce more energy to heal the damage and prepare for an increased demand. They use recovery time to respond to the stressor, which is why recovery is

## ROS: CELLULAR SMOKE SIGNALS

Hormesis at the mitochondrial level is called mitochondrial hormesis, or *mito-hormesis*. Because the mitochondria use a lot of oxygen, their energy production creates a waste product called reactive oxygen species, or ROS. You can think of these like cellular smoke signals that are good or bad, depending on the source. Many different processes in the body create ROS, including metabolism. Low levels can be hormetic, improving mitochondrial function through adaptation. Just like lower levels of stress improve resilience, lower levels of ROS strengthen rather than destroy mitochondria.[8] A number of studies have demonstrated that many of the hormetic activities biohackers use to increase physical and metabolic resilience also trigger mitohormesis through the production of ROS: calorie restriction, hypoxia (temporary oxygen deprivation), temperature stress, and exercise. As you experiment with biohacking your resilience with hormetic stressors, you are increasing the health and resilience of your mitochondria through mitohormesis.

But we also get ROS from outside the body, from exposure to pollution, alcohol, tobacco smoke, heavy metals, solvents, pesticides, high heat, ultraviolet light, overcooked meat and fat, and certain drugs.[9] You can think of these ROS as like the exhaust fumes from the action of a car engine. Ideally, they are neutralized by the body's antioxidant defenses,[10] but they have the potential to cause cellular damage. Eating a diet high in colorful fruits and vegetables as well as natural detoxifiers like spirulina and chlorella filled with natural anti-oxidants can mitigate some of this damage and help you thrive.

an important part of hormesis. With the right dose of exercise and sufficient recovery, weight lifting makes you stronger and more physically resilient. That's hormesis at work.

Here are some general examples of how to toggle between stress and recovery, to stimulate mitochondrial biogenesis. I'll tell you more about how to do these activities later, but for now, this chart demonstrates how you could expose yourself to potentially positive stressors followed by recovery.

## Toggling Mitohormetic Stressors

| STRESSOR | RECOVERY |
| --- | --- |
| Cold exposure / cold plunge | Heat / sauna |
| Fasting | Eating |
| Demanding work | Recovery |
| Sunlight exposure | Sleep (circadian rhythms) |
| HIIT (high-intensity interval training) | Rest days |
| Weight lifting | Massage or foam rolling |
| Eating low carb or dropping into ketosis (fat metabolism) | Raising your carbohydrate intake (carb metabolism) |
| Hypoxia (breath-holding) | Hyperoxia (breathwork, like deep breathing) |
| High pressure (HBOT, mountains, diving) | Normal atmospheric pressure (sea level) |
| Psychosocial stress | Play or quality time with loved ones |

As you can see, for every stressor, there is an opposite recovery action. This is a good way to think about stress: it's not bad if you get time to recover. Remember, the ability to *adapt to adversity* is at the core of robust health. Hormesis provides a simple method for promoting mitochondrial function and becoming more resilient. It teaches your body to adapt to adversity via the mitochondria.

But engaging with hormesis also requires that you pay attention to your body's subtle signals. If you do any of these stressors and feel like you're getting drained rather than energized, that means you aren't getting enough recovery. Hormesis requires that balance. You may need to pull back and focus solely on recovery until you heal and can endure more stress. Always remember that when demand exceeds capacity, the body breaks down. Don't emulate those biohackers who hit themselves so hard with stressors to get stronger that they cause long-term reduced resilience.

There is a famous quote from Friedrich Nietzsche, which seems to apply to hormesis: "What doesn't kill us makes us stronger." This line is often quoted in discussions about hormesis.[11] But please don't even come close to killing yourself! What doesn't kill us *does not* always make us stronger. I have some friends who are serious athletes who train aggressively all the time. When they got COVID, they developed serious long-haul symptoms. I believe their immune systems were impaired by their habit of extreme training without recovery. I also had a patient who was doing long sauna sessions followed by twenty-minute cold plunges. He developed major hypothalamic-pituitary-adrenal (HPA) axis dysfunction—a chronic stress condition that exhausts the adrenals and interferes with healthy cortisol output, causing many health issues, including chronic fatigue, depression, and frequent illness.

For women especially, I advise a minimum-effective-dose strategy when experimenting with hormesis. Extreme stressors can sometimes be strengthening if they don't last too long and you are already really strong, but it's easy to beat yourself down unintentionally, draining your batteries rather than increasing their capacity, and then you can get sick or injured. I can't tell you how many women I have seen overdo biohacking (often too much exercise and too much fasting or calorie restriction) and end up losing their periods, losing their hair, and burning out. One of my primary goals in writing this book is to help you find a balance between challenging yourself and *recovering*. Your period is a barometer of your health and if it stops, it's important that you re-examine your lifestyle and consider how you can nurture yourself back into balance.

Another side effect of too much biohacking combined with too much stress is the exacerbation or development of thyroid dysfunction. There are quite a lot of people with overt thyroid dysfunction or subclinical hypothyroidism who aren't aware of how important thyroid health is to mitochondrial function. Too much stress can put the female body in particular at risk by lowering thyroid hormone output as an adaptive response—this is a result of the body lowering metabolic rate to survive challenging times. In ancient times, this could help us survive a famine by lowering our caloric needs, but for a modern woman, it means she burns fewer calories, makes less body heat, and generally feels like crap. Thyroid hormones are profoundly influential on mitochondria, and low thyroid hormones will influence our metabolism like a thermostat. When you have low thyroid hormones, you're cold all the time and you can't lose weight no matter what you try. When your thyroid hormones are adequate, you're able to maintain a healthy body temperature and basal metabolic rate.

All that being said, when you *aren't* stressed, you can really dig into hormesis. A lot of my patients aren't necessarily in a state of chronic stress that's compromising their function. They can handle a lot of stress, and what they really want to do is become superhuman. In a culture of convenience and easy living, the person who has a body and mind capable of steely resilience against adversity really does seem like a superhero. If that sounds cool to you, then increasing your resilience with hormesis (*after* getting chronic stress states under control) could be your training ground. Here are some ways to use hormesis to signal your mitochondria to make more energy.

## Mitohormetic Stress Interventions to Try

First, I need to mention that you do not and should not employ all these mitohormetic stressors at once. That's a recipe for allostatic overload, aka stressing your system so much that you do more harm than good. The first thing to ask yourself is: What is my health condition right now? I have made the mistake of doing fasting and HIIT training on top of major life stressors and it really drained my capacity. But, at other times, I've been strong and recovered, and experienced astonishing health gains from these practices. If you are burned out or under enormous stress, extra stress is not going to help you thrive. You may need months of recovery to get back into a place of strength.

In general though, even when you are in good baseline health, it's best to practice these interventions one at a time, to gain the adaptations you are aiming for. Once you feel stronger, you can add more, always listening to your body to see if you can handle the extra challenge. Think about where you want to get stronger first. If you are intolerant to cold, working on cold adaptation for a few months will build your resilience to cold. If you are metabolically inflexible, practicing ketosis for a month can help you become fat adapted. Intermittent fasting can help you get better at going without food. Weight lifting can build your physical resilience.

When you've got your first target, try your hormetic stressor one or two times a week at most until you notice you are getting stronger and the stressor is feeling less stressful. For the most part, less is more when layering different stressors. A typical regimen might be to do a sauna and cold plunge one to two days a week and weight training three to four days a week.

I've devoted whole sections of this book to biohacking movement, metabolism (food), and stress, but here are some specific ways to practice hormesis that aren't included in those sections:

- HYPOXIA. Hypoxia, or lack of oxygen, triggers the kidneys to make more EPO (erythropoietin), a hormone that increases your red blood cell mass to enhance the red blood cells' ability to transport oxygen to the mitochondria. This is particularly good for people who are looking to improve their endurance training performance.

There are a few ways you can do this.

FIRST IS THROUGH exercising at high altitudes (e.g., going skiing or snowboarding or hiking at higher elevations). Some research suggests to get the full benefits, you have to be at a higher altitude for at least three weeks. Some hard-core biohackers and athletes sleep in an altitude tent to get these benefits.

THE SECOND WAY IS with breathwork practices like Wim Hoff breathing, which combines periods of hyperventilation with breath holds. Ari Whitten of the Energy Blueprint[12] has a slightly less strenuous method that entails walking at a normal pace, holding your breath for as many steps as you can while counting your steps (don't hold it so long that you get faint or light-headed), and then breathing normally until you catch your breath again. He recommends repeating this four to twelve times.

THE THIRD WAY IS to use resisted breathing using an elevation training mask combined with HIIT training or steady-state aerobic exercise. You can also wear these masks while sedentary, five minutes on, five minutes off, monitoring your oxygen saturation level (SpO$_2$) with a finger pulse oximeter and aiming to get your oxygen level down to 85 percent.

- HYPEROXIA. HBOT (hyperbaric oxygen therapy) is a type of hyperoxia that pushes oxygen into your tissues while you are in a high-pressure hyperbaric chamber. This therapy can be expensive and time consuming, but it's good for people recovering from injury, infection, or chronic illnesses like viral infections. Oxygen can improve immune function and enhance oxygen delivery to the tissues to speed healing. Some athletes use it to enhance recovery, and frequent travelers may do HBOT sessions after long-term travel to fight jet lag. Biohackers sometimes buy their own in-home units and answer email inside the chamber. Typically, for healing purposes, do ninety-minute sessions five days a week for twenty to thirty treatments.

- **COLD PLUNGES/COLD WATER IMMERSION.** Start with cold showers. This will build your resilience to cold. Work your way up to being in the shower for two to three minutes without turning it off.

  IF YOU LIVE BY A LAKE OR COLD BODY OF WATER, you can do a cold plunge that way (as long as you can swim, of course). Polar plunges are popular in colder climates. If you don't have a body of water to dip into, you can fill your bathtub with ice or you can buy a freezer, fill it with water, turn it on, and climb in for a DIY cold plunge. There are companies that produce high-end cold-plunge tubs for home use as well.

  IF YOU ARE NEW TO COLD PLUNGES, aim for around fifty to sixty degrees Fahrenheit. Before you get into the water, center yourself with your breath so you don't hyperventilate when you get in. You need to stay immersed for at least a minute to trigger the beneficial adaptations, ideally two to three minutes. Try to slow down your breathing so each breath takes three seconds. Slower breathing trains your nervous system to relax under stress.

- **HEAT/SAUNA.** If you have access to a sauna, I recommend using it twice a week for best results, ideally at a temperature of at least 174 degrees Fahrenheit for at least twenty minutes. A sauna can be a replacement for exercise for those who are sidelined by injury or chronic disease (always get cleared to use a sauna by your doctor first). Evidence suggests sauna use activates heat shock proteins, which helps prevent muscle atrophy and preserves muscle mass.[13]

By now you have mastered the most challenging part of the book. You've learned about how the mitochondria work, which is to say you have learned how the batteries in your cells work, and how you can strengthen them and grow more of them through hormesis. You've also grasped what may be one of the largest paradigm shifts in medicine

## STRESSED PLANTS THAT MAKE YOU STRONGER

When plants undergo environmental stressors such as extreme temperature or lack of adequate water, they produce stress-induced compounds that are intended to protect them from predators. Certain plant chemicals found in nature are actually beneficial in small doses to the animals and humans that eat them. This phenomenon is known as xenohormesis, and eating these plants is a mitohormetic stressor that can make you stronger.

The human body has evolved mechanisms for detoxifying what we eat to protect us,[14] so when we ingest these compounds, enzymes in the liver are stimulated to rapidly detoxify and excrete them, improving the body's ability to detoxify in general. These plant compounds also activate our adaptive stress response, inducing antioxidant enzymes and cell survival proteins, while inhibiting inflammatory pathways. If you never ate anything remotely toxic, your liver would downregulate detoxification enzymes and wouldn't have an adaptive anti-inflammatory stress response to plants because it would determine you didn't need this. But little bits of toxins cue the liver to adapt and release these enzymes. This is how xenohormetic stressors ultimately reduce inflammation and generate protective antioxidants and detoxifiers.

Some examples of these low-dose toxins that have a beneficial effect[15] are the sulforaphane found in broccoli sprouts, the curcumin found in turmeric, epicatechins in green tea, polyphenols in coffee, and flavanols in cacao. I like to take these in concentrated form, as elixirs. Some of my favorites are golden milk with turmeric and black pepper, matcha lattes made with almond milk and maca, and spicy ceremonial cacao made with cacao paste and cayenne pepper.

Another way to take advantage of xenohormesis is through foraging. Wild plants are full of these toxins, even more so than farmed produce. I like to forage in any new environment. During the summer of 2020, I foraged for morel mushrooms, fiddlehead ferns, mulberries, marionberries, and ramps. Recently I found chanterelle mushrooms—I was so proud! Just make sure you learn from an experienced forager so you can learn to avoid poisonous mushrooms and other poisonous plants.

happening today: a movement toward a new way of seeing the body through the lens of energy. By optimizing your lifestyle to cultivate energy effectively and challenging yourself to master new techniques that enhance physiologic resilience, you can become more adaptable to demands and you can begin to see the body as a dynamic system perfectly designed to help you survive in a complex world.

## MITOCHONDRIA-PROMOTING BIOHACKS IN THIS CHAPTER

### For chronic fatigue or long-haul COVID-19

- Lymphatic drainage: sweating, dry brushing, self-massage, foam rolling, walking, yoga
- Respiratory training and cough exercises
- Anti-inflammatory diet rich in colorful vegetables, fruit, legumes, fatty fish, spices, nuts, and seeds, and low in refined grains and processed food
- Ozone therapy
- Hyperbaric oxygen therapy
- Anti-inflammatory supplements: vitamin D with vitamins $K_1$ and $K_2$, melatonin at night, curcumin, pharmaceutical grade fish oil.
- Mitochondrial function enhancers: magnesium, acetyl-L carnitine, pyrroloquinoline, and coenzyme $Q_{10}$.
- Electrolytes, or a pinch of Himalayan sea salt in water

### For lung support

- NAC
- Vitamin C
- Mullein

### For preventing blood clots

- Nattokinase
- Serratiopeptidase enzymes
- High-dose pharmaceutical-grade omega-3s

*For brain fog*

- Desiccated grass-fed New Zealand beef brain
- High-dose, pharmaceutical-grade omega-3s

*For detoxification*

- Liposomal glutathione
- Binders like activated charcoal, bentonite clay, modified citrus pectin, and chlorella
- Filter your water and air at home

*For boosting mitochondrial health and significantly reducing the risk of chronic diseases*

- Quit smoking
- Eat a nutrient-rich, plant-centric diet
- Exercise regularly
- Achieve or maintain a healthy body weight
- Minimize alcohol consumption

*To practice hormesis, toggle between . . .*

- Cold exposure/cold plunge and heat/sauna
- Fasting and feasting
- Demanding work and recovery
- Sunlight exposure and sleep
- HIIT or cardiovascular training workouts and rest
- Weight lifting and massage or foam rolling
- Fasting/ketosis (fat metabolism) and refeeding (carb metabolism)
- Hypoxia (breath-holding) and hyperoxia (breathwork, like deep breathing)
- High pressure/mountains/diving/hyperbaric oxygen chambers and normal pressure
- Psychosocial stress and play or quality time with friends
- For xenohormesis, eat more plants, especially wild foraged plants

# CHAPTER 3

# The Quantified Self

## BIOHACKING TO CREATE HEALTH

Biohacking is the process of applying cutting-edge scientific knowledge using N = 1 experiments to become the healthiest versions of ourselves—mind, body, and spirit.

— Molly Maloof

A lot of us exist on autopilot. We live day-to-day, doing what's expected, following the rules, eating what others eat, moving like others move, working like others work. Often we don't even realize that just about everything we do is influenced by powerful forces in society designed to lure us into consuming hyper-palatable foods, using hyper-convenient transportation, and absorbing hyper-stressful content.

Biohacking means shutting off the autopilot. It means bringing conscious awareness to what you do and how it affects your body and mind, then using what you learn to make changes—whether they are simple or complex, low-tech or high-tech—to heal and optimize your biology. It's about noticing, maintaining, and repairing when necessary. It means recognizing, in your complex body, when something doesn't feel right, before it can turn into a big problem, and it means solving problems you already have with things you can do yourself.

Habit change is hard, but biohacking is a way to achieve it because it takes habits off autopilot. It gives you a method (self-knowledge through observation, measurement, and tracking) and tools (lab tests, practices, interventions, and ways to monitor progress) to change them.

Your body is your home, and its entire purpose is to serve and protect you. We're all born with internal sensors that alert us to problems, but we've forgotten how to hear the alarms that go off when those sensors detect something is wrong. Biohacking offers us a way to turn up the volume and interpret the messages. But biohacking is not a quick-fix process. It's about the small things you do every day that accumulate. Real, lasting health is about slow, sustained habit formation and consistency over time.

I've already shown you some ways to start biohacking, and you may already be doing more biohacking than you realize, but if you really want to join the ranks of biohackers worldwide—especially the rapidly growing community of women biohackers out there—then it can help to get a little more context about what biohacking really is. Many people have misconceptions about biohacking, so let's take a closer look at what this seemingly modern "trend" is really all about.

## Biohacking Isn't New

There is a misconception that biohacking is high-tech. It can be, but it doesn't have to be. It can be expensive, too, but it doesn't have to be. It's something humans have been doing all along to survive. Calling it "biohacking" is new, but the solution-oriented, survival-oriented, health-improving nature of biohacking is as old as humans.

Biohacking has helped us, and can continue to help us, progress as a species. Yes, there are ways to track and test and measure that we haven't always had access to, and there are still some high-tech gadgets that are out of reach for many of us, but the old ways (like meditation, breathing practices, intermittent fasting and ketosis, cold exposure, and tracking the menstrual cycle) are often as useful as, if not more useful than, the new ways (such as continuous glucose monitoring, $VO_2$ max tracking, heart rate variability monitoring, step tracking, blood oxygen measuring, and so much more). Fortunately, you have access to both. There are plenty of interventions that are free or cost very little, but any investment you do make will pay for itself over time as you reap the enhanced health, productivity, and performance benefits biohacking offers.

At its heart, biohacking is based on viewing the body as a system of systems. Quantifying the self through biohacking helps you get to know your body in all its complexity by understanding how your lifestyle affects the different systems in your body. Your digestive system, endocrine system, reproductive system, musculoskeletal system, brain, and cardiovascular system can all be hacked for better healing as well as for optimization.

## Biohacking Can Help You Achieve Goals

What you want to achieve will largely determine how you will start biohacking. Are you trying to balance your hormones to minimize PMS or get pregnant? Are you trying to improve your physical or mental performance? Are you trying to build better immunity to avoid getting sick? Are you trying to get rid of your acid reflux, your sore knee, or your brain fog? Whatever it is, there are things you can do to tweak your biology so it does what you want it to do. You don't have to be a genius, a billionaire, or a scientist. All you have to do is have the desire to get to know your body better and get the most you can out of it, for as long as possible.

Part of biohacking is gathering information. For instance, you could get a lab test to measure your vitamin D, to see if you are deficient, which could be impacting your immune health, hormone balance, and blood sugar control. Vitamin D deficiency happens at less than 20 ng/mL, insufficiency happens at less than 30 ng/mL, and optimal vitamin D levels are 50–80 ng/mL. Roughly 42 percent of the U.S.

population is vitamin D deficient. Knowing this number and keeping track of how it responds to things you do, like getting more sunshine or taking supplements, is biohacking.

Biohacking can also help you determine whether the objective data you gather (like heart rate, blood sugar level, or sleep quality) matches your subjective assessments about yourself (whether you feel anxious or calm, hungry or satisfied, energetic or tired) and what it means when they don't match. You might be amazed at how much you can learn about how your body works. For example, anyone who's ever been hungry and gotten into a fight before dinner with someone they care about has experienced being "hangry." Hunger coupled with anger is a negative internal signal that's easy to misinterpret. You think your significant other is purposefully aggravating you, when really, you just need to eat. Wearing a continuous glucose monitor can show you that low blood sugar is the real problem. (It can also provide a ton of information about what foods are best for you to eat and how you respond to other lifestyle changes—I'll tell you more about how to use one in chapter 7.)

## Biohacking Is for Women

Biohacking originated in the Bay Area technology scene, which is male dominated, and, like technology, the biohacking field has been dominated by men. When I first started going to biohacking events, I was often one of a handful of women there. It was a boys' club.

But biohacking has never *really* been a male sport, if you consider who is actually doing it beyond who has the most popular podcasts or social media accounts. I believe women were the original biohackers. We had to be. Otherwise, our hormonal cycles, from puberty to menopause, would have interfered with our functioning and even our survival. We couldn't just take a week off every month. No, we had to keep going, giving birth to and raising children, finding and cooking food, solving problems, bringing communities together, and doing everything else women have been doing at every stage of human evolution, even when we are tired, cranky, breastfeeding, or bleeding. So, we figured it out, in low-tech ways, as well as we could.

Look at what people have been doing for thousands of years, since before anybody ever thought to call it biohacking, and you will see that it has always been something women have done. Women track their bodies' hormonal cycles, fertility, postpartum changes, and menopause. We may try to optimize fertility or prevent breast cancer. We want to know what's wrong, and why, and how to fix it, so we can fix ourselves and others. We are often more body-aware, more tuned into our own health needs and those of our families, and more vigilant about repairing and preserving health than our male peers.

Women also go to the doctor more often than men. We interact with the healthcare system to get birth control, do preventive screenings, and get help for polycystic ovary syndrome (PCOS), fibroids, endometriosis, fertility, pregnancy, miscarriage, hormone replacement therapy, and more. In general, we tend to be highly attuned to and invested in our health.

Most of the popular literature about biohacking has been produced by men, and most of the trendy high-tech tools and techniques for biohacking have been created by men, which means that to a large extent, they are engineered to work with men's bodies, not women's. For that matter, even traditional medical research is still primarily conducted with male test groups, and the results of that research are not always applicable to women. Women are harder and more expensive to study because of their cycles.

But cycles are exactly why the way guys biohack doesn't always work for us; we have hormonal and physiological differences, and, importantly, different biological imperatives, from an evolutionary standpoint. A body made for the challenges of pregnancy and caretaking has very different needs from a body made for the challenges of hunting and battle. As nutrition scientist and exercise physiologist Stacy Sims says, "You are not a small man. Stop eating and training like one."[1]

## HORMONES AND GENDER CONSIDERATIONS

As much as I see the benefits of eliminating gender roles in society—and I believe it is a human right to change or be without gender—biologically, there are differences in the bodies of people born male or born female. Biologically and biochemically, we have different experiences, and biohacking is largely subject to the hormonal milieu. But these can be hacked, too. Trans people are some of the most forward-thinking, radical biohackers, in my opinion—they are changing their bodies and entire hormonal environments to change their genders.

Ketogenic diets are a good example of how male-dominated bio-hacking doesn't work as well for women. A lot of women find that the ketogenic diet (very high fat, very low carb) works well for a few months but then begins to make them feel worse or leads to weight gain. There are some women who thrive on a keto diet, but more often than not, the continuous ketogenic diet ultimately ends up feeling wrong to many women. It's not that ketosis (burning fat instead of sugar) is a bad state to be in. It's just that women, especially when they are in their fertile years, need more carbs than men and respond better to cyclical ketosis, or what is sometimes called carb cycling (alternating periods of lower carb and higher carb eating) according to their menstrual cycles—especially in women who are athletic. The menstrual cycle causes a woman's energy to change dramatically over the course of four weeks, which means that your body processes food, performs physically, and handles stress differently depending on where you are in your cycle. One week, keto might be just what you need. The next week, not so much. The cyclical nature of a woman's biology is a better match for cyclical diets and cyclical exercise in general.

Of course, our bodies and our hormonal makeups also evolve throughout our lives. We are biochemically four different people (at least) throughout each month, during each phase of our cycle, and also throughout different periods of our lives—childhood, adolescence, young adulthood, our fertile years, pregnancy, postpartum, menopause, and postmenopause. Men generally have just three phases of their lives—childhood, adulthood, and senior years—and fairly consistent hormonal profiles during these phases (depending on whether or not they intervene with hormone replacement).

When it comes to weight change, whether you are trying to lose some or gain some (altering your body weight on purpose is biohacking), women need a more nuanced approach than just calories in, calories out, because our hormones affect our metabolism. This is why men often lose weight more easily than women. Men have a tendency to try to force their bodies into different states with extreme protocols, like fasting or long-term keto or calorie restriction. This often works pretty well for them, but women's bodies are much more sensitive to nutrient deprivation because of our biological imperatives. When a woman deprives herself of food (such as through fasting or a ketogenic diet), it can downshift her metabolic rate. That's an adaptive response—if there weren't food available and you needed to nourish a baby, a slower metabolic rate would help ensure your and the baby's survival. We respond better to gentle shifts rather than muscling through.

This all makes sense from an evolutionary perspective. Our primitive genetics are designed for men to hunt and gather under extreme conditions. They might have to fight off predatory animals or survive in the wild without food for long periods without losing the energy to hunt. Women, by contrast, had to be prepared for more extreme internal conditions, like pregnancy.

Interestingly, postmenopausal women can take on more metabolic stress and thrive on it better than a younger woman can because their bodies no longer "worry" about pregnancy. As long as they are healthy and not under a lot of emotional stress, they often have better luck with more extended ketogenic diets and longer periods of fasting, as well as more intense exercise. This is helpful since, as we get older, we naturally become less insulin sensitive, which can make weight gain easier and weight loss harder.

Beyond biological differences between men and women, there are of course cultural forces at work. For instance, women are more likely to develop eating disorders, like binge eating or orthorexia (an obsession with "perfect" eating). We have been steeped in diet culture and also in a culture that prioritizes a woman's attractiveness over other qualities. All this can influence how and especially why we may choose to bio-hack.

Whatever your goals, biohacking can help you leverage your hormonal fluctuations, increasing brain power, improving sleep quality, and actually providing benefits from stress through hormesis. You can learn when to do things that take a lot of effort and when to schedule more downtime, based on your biological cycles and your body's own wisdom. You can improve your health, self-confidence, personal success, and relationships. You can have a mind-blowing sex life—and a safe one, too. You can learn how to access happiness, contentment, and joy, and you can reconnect with not only your own biology but the biology and ecology of the natural world, which operates in cycles, just like women do.

## How to Start Biohacking

I'm going to give you all kinds of tools and methods for biohacking throughout this book, but first, let's make a plan to examine and intervene in your health systematically. In my practice and in the course

## BIOHACKING CAN FUEL ORTHOREXIA

Biohacking can actually worsen orthorexia because women can become obsessive about tracking every aspect of nutrition, calories, exercise, and weight, and can develop anxiety if the numbers ever go in the wrong direction. Similar disorders are orthosomnia, an obsession with getting the "perfect" sleep that has been associated with the use of sleep-tracking devices,[2] and exercise obsession, which can be a product of tracking apps that tally calories burned, time spent exercising, steps taken, etc. This is something to watch out for when you start tracking. If you know you are susceptible to obsessive behavior, you should avoid getting too focused on quantified data. Instead, stay in tune with your own reactions, stay alert to any signs of obsessiveness or anxiety, and biohack *like a woman,* with respect for your body's individual cycles and changing energy needs and capacity.

I teach at Stanford, and I outline a health optimization process based on the scientific method. Remember, the idea of biohacking is to turn off autopilot and become more aware of what's going on internally, so you can stop engaging in energy-draining behaviors and start creating habits around energy-enhancing behaviors. Following is a graphic I use to explain my recommended health optimization process for biohacking.

STEP 1: IDENTIFY. First, it's important to get clear on your goals and motivations. Maybe your goal is to improve your blood sugar or get stronger. Maybe you're motivated to improve your health so you have more energy to do the things you love or you want to balance your hormones to benefit your fertility. You can think about this on your own, make some notes, or do some journaling to really get clear on what your goals are. You may have many goals and motivations, so it's a good idea to decide what you want to address first, or make a top-three list.

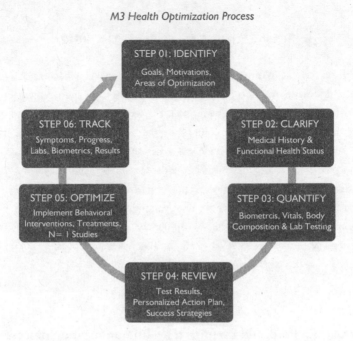

*M3 Health Optimization Process*

STEP 01: IDENTIFY
Goals, Motivations, Areas of Optimization

STEP 02: CLARIFY
Medical History & Functional Health Status

STEP 03: QUANTIFY
Biometrcis, Vitals, Body Composition & Lab Testing

STEP 04: REVIEW
Test Results, Personalized Action Plan, Success Strategies

STEP 05: OPTIMIZE
Implement Behavioral Interventions, Treatments, N= 1 Studies

STEP 06: TRACK
Symptoms, Progress, Labs, Biometrics, Results

**STEP 2: CLARIFY.** Next, look into your own health history, your family history, and your current state of health. Make a list of all the health issues in your family, and underline the issues that you are concerned you might develop or already have developed. Then frankly assess your subjective feelings about your own health. How healthy are you, if you had to guess? Think about your vulnerabilities (like a genetic predisposition to a health condition or something you're already showing signs of). Your vulnerabilities can become a place of strength if you decide to prioritize them. For example, chronic digestive problems are worth addressing because you eat food every day and it plays such a big role in your energy levels. Or if you have a family history of diabetes, you might want to zero in on blood sugar control.

**STEP 3: QUANTIFY.** A big part of biohacking is measuring. Measure your vital signs: heart rate, temperature, weight, blood pressure. Ask your doctor for some basic labs, if you can (see my website for a list of the top twenty labs you can get from your regular doctor, to get a baseline analysis of where your health is right now). Getting a body composition test can tell you if you have a high amount of visceral fat. Using a continuous glucose monitor can reveal whether you have blood sugar problems. Wearing a smartwatch can show you how many steps and how much sleep you are getting. Establishing baseline measurements will help you notice if the markers change over time. (I'll discuss these tools and interventions in more detail throughout the rest of this book.)

STEP 4: REVIEW. Once you have clarity on your goals, motivations, and risk factors, and you have some basic numbers, you can get a more objective perspective on your level of health and what is most urgent to focus on. Review what you've learned and make a plan of action personalized for you. I suggest keeping all this information in one place so you can refer back to it often, and so you can keep track of how your metrics change in response to changes in your lifestyle.

If you are younger (under thirty), use youth to your advantage. The habits you create today will carry into the years when hormones shift. Take care of yourself now so you don't have to spend your later life trying to fix your health.

If you're over thirty, you probably already have some entrenched habits that aren't serving you or your health, and those can be difficult to break. You probably also have a lot of competing demands on your time and resources. At this stage it takes more effort to change, but your commitment will pay off when you have more energy and resilience.

If you are over fifty and already in a stage of hormonal transition, just keep in mind that it is *never too late* to start increasing cellular energy production. Listen to what your body is telling you about how it

## THE VALUE OF LAB TESTS

I know that people don't like to buy a book and then read about more things they have to pay for, and I am not going to tell you that you absolutely have to invest in lab testing. However, if you really want to biohack your body, there are some things you will want to know about yourself that you can learn only from lab tests. Labs aren't just for diagnosing. In biohacking, they're tools that can help us better understand how our individual bodies function, and they're pretty fundamental for helping you shift your efforts in the right direction. They also help increase self-awareness. When you get the objective information that something is off, you can begin to learn how to feel it for yourself.

On my website, I list comprehensive labs for different purposes, from basic tests I think everyone should get (and that your doctor will probably be willing to order for you) to more complex labs you may need to get from a functional medicine doctor (see the Institute for Functional Medicine website to find one[3]), with panels for different purposes, depending on what you're working on. I've included information on what the labs are for and what the results mean, not just in terms of "normal" or "abnormal" but in terms of "optimal," so you know what to shoot for. Because tech companies are responding to demand, there are also many basic labs you can order and do on your own, without a doctor.

is changing with age, and get a feel for which changes seem okay and which ones don't. There are many aspects of so-called natural aging that really are not natural at all, nor necessary, and you can hack them.

STEP 5: OPTIMIZE. This step is where you implement your action plan. This may include changing habits, adding supplements, getting treatments, or making dietary shifts. The key to optimization is healthy habit formation. In the subsequent sections in this book, I will guide you toward ideals, and you can choose the habits you want to take on and the things you want to stop doing. The changes you make today can help you age better and increase your healthspan.

STEP 6: TRACK. It's important to close the loop that starts with goals and ends with action by monitoring any changes or improvements in your symptoms, labs, biomarkers, or other results of experimentation. This is how you find out what's working for you and what isn't. Then you can begin the process all over again with new goals and new intentions for optimizing different aspects of your health.

## You Can Start with Tracking

Although it's the final step in the system above, tracking can be a great place to dip your toe into biohacking. If you can measure something, you can change it. I challenge you to consider what you want for your health and life today, then to pick one thing to start tracking. Begin recording or journaling so you can get some perspective on how your lifestyle affects whatever you are tracking.

You might already be doing this, in which case you can begin doing it more purposefully or with more thoughtfulness around it. Maybe you have a smartwatch and you keep track of your steps. That's biohacking. Maybe you keep a food diary. That's biohacking. Maybe you use a period tracker, so your period doesn't surprise you every month. Biohacking. Maybe you track your exercise performance. That's biohacking, too.

What you decide to track depends on where you want to make an impact. If you want to start eating better, start tracking your food. If you want to start exercising more, start tracking your steps and workouts. If you want to get your hormones regulated, monitor for perimenopause, or track fertility, start tracking your menstrual cycle. We will learn more advanced ways to hack all of these aspects of health, but you can start now just by writing down what you eat, recording your workouts, using a pedometer, and/or keeping track of your period symptoms.

It's also important to understand that tracking isn't meant to be forever. The more you track and tune in, the more you will learn what those numbers *feel* like, and eventually, when good habits are in place, you won't need to track anymore. For instance, because I have used a continuous glucose monitor so often, I know what it feels like when my blood sugar is too high or too low. Sometimes I'll put on a monitor again for a couple of weeks to check in, but generally, I can tell when I need to eat something because my blood sugar is low, adjust what I'm eating when it's borderline, or get in a cardio session when I need to bring my blood sugar back down fast.

## Creating a Routine

Years ago, I kept a long list of the health practices I aimed to do every day. It was super ambitious, as I was trying to intervene into a lot of different parts of my life. Today, my list is much shorter. I recommend making a list for your morning and evening routines. These can anchor

| A.M. | P.M. |
| --- | --- |
| Wake up | Stop eating around six or seven P.M. |
| Visualization or intention setting | Wind down around eight P.M. |
| 5 minutes of breathwork | Recovery practices (PEMF, yin yoga, acupressure mat, massage gun, or infrared mat) |
| 15 minutes of meditation | |
| Brush teeth | |
| Drink water | Wash face, moisturize |
| Make coffee, tea, or elixir | Brush teeth, tongue scrape, floss |
| Eat small snack before workout | P.M. supplements |
| Exercise and stretching | Read |
| Shower, makeup, get dressed | Visualize, meditate, or pray |
| A.M. supplements | Sleep |
| Organize my day | |

your day and your health. Above are things I do as part of my morning and evening routines (note that I don't always get everything on these lists done every day). Feel free to pick and choose a few things from my lists that might fit your schedule and lifestyle.

The more you learn, the more you can create checklists and routines for yourself, and the more those checklists and routines can evolve as you create new habits and make new goals. The ultimate goal of bio-hacking is to gain intrinsic knowledge and motivation to be healthy and have mastery of and autonomy over your life. With practice and commitment, you can learn to naturally, instinctively, and intuitively live in a way that is best for your body. But until you get to that point, let's focus on creating your transformation incrementally, one hack at a time.

### BIOHACKS IN THIS CHAPTER

- Identify what your health goals and motivations are. In what areas are you hoping to improve your health? In what ways would you like to optimize?

- Assess your medical history, family history, and subjective feeling about your current health status.

- Measure your vitals and get basic labs to get a quantitative view of your current health status.

- Make a personal action plan: What do you want to tackle first? What strategies do you want to try?

- Start implementing some simple behavioral changes in the areas you have prioritized for improvement.

- Track what you are working on (like logging food, steps, or exercise minutes, monitoring your blood sugar, etc.) to see and measure your progress.

- Create a morning and evening routine for your day, to help you tackle your goals more systematically.

# PART II

# MAKING MORE BATTERIES

# CHAPTER 4

# Movement Is Life's Energy Signal

*Diseases fly from the presence of a person habituated to regular physical exercise.*

—Susruta, 600 BCE

If there is one way to build more cellular batteries, it is to exercise regularly. Exercise uses energy, but it also triggers the creation of more energy, increasing energy capacity and providing you with ample stores of energy to use in whatever way you want. The more you move, the brighter your spark. This is exercise 101.

And yet, physical activity is at a low point.[1] According to a Surgeon General's Report,[2] over 60 percent of U.S. adults don't get the recommended amount of activity, and 25 percent are not active *at all*. According to the American Physiological Society, 85 percent of the 325 million people in the U.S. get less than the U.S. government and World Health Organization guidelines for daily physical activity required for health.[3] Average daily sitting time has increased from around an hour to eight hours for teens and almost six and a half hours for adults[4]—but often much more for those who work at full-time desk jobs and have long commutes.[5] We live in a culture of knowledge workers who sit in front of computers all day, so it's easy to become sedentary and not even notice. That's one significant reason why 88 percent of Americans are metabolically unhealthy.[6]

The standards for being classified as physically inactive are: getting less than 60 minutes a day of moderate- or vigorous-intensity aerobic activity for five- to seventeen-year-olds, and less than 150 minutes a week of moderate- or vigorous-intensity aerobic exercise for adults age eighteen and above. That seems like a lot to some people, but it's really a minimal amount of movement when you consider how we are built. We are genetically designed to move at moderate intensity throughout our day.

According to evolutionary biology, about two million years ago, climate change forced humans to move from forests to more open habitats, and to shift their diets from eating like chimps to hunting and gathering. That required us to move our bodies at a moderate intensity over long periods with high levels of aerobic activity, enabling us to develop spatial navigation, better motor control, and improved memory, attention, and executive function.[7] Basically, our ancestors were cognitively engaged endurance athletes foraging to survive, which led to enhanced neural responses to exercise and the necessity to move in a lot of different ways.

Since the 1950s, researchers have been wondering, and worrying, about sedentary behavior. One study of bus drivers from 1953 showed that those who were sedentary had twice the rate of heart disease as those who were physically active.[8] If you look at the health of people living in Amish societies without modern transportation or conveniences like electrical appliances, you can glimpse the impact of technology on the body—the Amish walk around sixteen thousand steps a day on average, while the average American walks around five thousand steps a day.[9] It's certainly easier to move less, but we are paying a price.

## The Health Risks of a Sedentary Lifestyle

Being sedentary is more dangerous than being overweight. People with low cardiorespiratory fitness are more likely to die from lack of fitness than they are from having a high BMI (body mass index).[10] A sedentary lifestyle decreases mitochondrial density in the cells, which equates to less energy production and early exhaustion. Remember that exercise signals the mitochondria to get stronger. A sedentary life does the opposite. If your mitochondria don't think you need much energy, they won't produce it. Even a vigorous workout at the gym can be essentially canceled out if you go on to sit all day afterward. Constant sitting can also cause slumping, contributing to reduced lung volume and an inability to get a really deep breath. This can impair focus and concentration, not to mention lung capacity.[11]

Sitting has metabolic effects on skeletal muscle and fat tissue as well. The body stops breaking down fat into energy for muscles to use because the muscles aren't using it.[12] Instead, it keeps the fat in storage. Technically, what's happening is that a fat-burning enzyme called lipoprotein lipase decreases as activity decreases. One of the benefits of just standing to do your work (such as with a standing desk) is that you can increase the amount of lipoprotein lipase your body is releasing,[13] which can help to keep your muscles from ending up fatty and deconditioned.

Sitting is associated with risks like obesity, metabolic syndrome, diabetes, depression, anxiety, and heart disease.[14] The heart is full of mitochondria, so it makes sense that sedentary behavior could lead to a higher risk of heart failure, which is what happens when your heart no longer has the energy to pump. If you really want to have a nice strong heart, you must send the signals for the heart to make more mitochondria, so it has more energy it can use to stay strong and functional. To send those signals, you have to move. Think about hormesis: stressors with recovery trigger more energy output. Cardiovascular exercise is a hormetic stressor for the heart and lungs.

Prolonged sitting also increases cancer risk. A study published in *JAMA Oncology* found that sedentary people had an 82 percent higher risk of dying from cancer compared to the least sedentary people.[15]

Even when people meet the guidelines for physical activity, prolonged sedentary behavior still increases the chances of premature death. You can work out all you want, but if you sit all day long after working out, it still increases the risk of early death.[16] Going to the gym is really important, but it doesn't attenuate the risk associated with spending all day sitting in front of a screen.

But you can reverse all these health-damaging conditions, and you don't even have to go to the gym, necessarily. You can do it through

## ACCELEROMETERS

An accelerometer is a device that measures acceleration, which is a way to measure movement. This is a biohacking device that can give you a reality check about how much you are actually moving. A study comparing how much physical activity people *estimated* they got to how much they *actually* got using an accelerometer showed that people generally overestimate how much activity they get during the day. While 12.5 percent of people in the study self-reported getting no physical activity, the accelerometer showed that 53 percent of people got no physical activity. While 62 percent of people reported getting sufficient physical activity, according to the accelerometer, only 9.6 percent achieved sufficient physical activity.[17]

Until you slap one of these things on your wrist, you probably won't really know how you're doing. Smartwatches and other fitness wearables generally contain accelerometers and measure step count and movement, so you might already be wearing one. I had a patient who suffered from migraines, and when I asked him how much exercise he got, he told me that he didn't exercise. I told him to get a fitness tracker to measure his steps, and it turned out he was getting only about a thousand steps a day. The recommendation is ten thousand steps, which is the equivalent of about five miles. He didn't realize how little he was moving until he saw the number. That gave him the motivation to change. He started exercising more, slowly adding one thousand steps at time, and with this increase in exercise, along with dietary changes to improve his blood sugar regulation and supplements like magnesium, his migraines resolved.

NEAT, which stands for "non-exercise activity thermogenesis." This is the most basic way to begin moving and breaking the cycle of sedentary living.

## NEAT = Everyday Movement

"Non-exercise activity thermogenesis" is a fancy way of describing the energy you expend to do everything during the day that is not sleeping, eating, or purposeful exercise (like sports and running or gym workouts). NEAT is achieved by just walking around, running to catch the bus, doing yard work, cleaning, even fidgeting.[18] This activity can add up significantly throughout the day.

You may often hear that exercise, while good for you, doesn't impact weight loss much. That's true, but what does impact weight loss is NEAT activity. The reason is that how you move throughout the day contributes to a lot more energy usage than a single exercise session. When you move, your mitochondria get the signal to produce more energy, not just during your exercise time but all day long.

### THE CONNECTION BETWEEN MOVING AND EATING

Spontaneous movement isn't necessarily spontaneous. It's an instinct based on energy intake.[19] The natural human (and animal) tendency is to move more in response to eating more, and to move less in response to eating less.

The problem is that we have overridden this instinct because of how easy it is to overeat and how easy it is not to move in our current culture, but you can start to counter this mismatch between movement and energy intake by purposefully moving more. If you never sit for long periods of time, moving your body at least every thirty minutes or so throughout the day, you can get back into sync with your appetite cues.

Also, NEAT counteracts the hazardous effect of being sedentary. Moving throughout the day uses up the ATP your mitochondria are producing and minimizes a buildup of that cellular exhaust (ROS) that is a byproduct of energy production. Doing NEAT activities is like opening the garage door to let the exhaust fumes out and taking the car out for a drive. We want our "car" to be driving around (moving, living), not sitting in the garage. We need to use our fuel.

## Track Your Steps

A simple biohack for beginning to monitor how much you move around during the day is step tracking. Smartwatches, smartphones, and inexpensive pedometers are all ways to track your steps, to see if you're moving around enough. Begin by measuring how many steps you take on average. Track your steps for a week to see where you land. This will give you an idea of your activity level. There are many different opinions about how much is enough, but after doing a lot of research, I devised a simple system:

SEDENTARY: Less than 5,000 steps per day

LOW ACTIVE: 5,000 to 7,500 steps per day

ACTIVE: 7,500 to 11,000 steps per day

VERY ACTIVE: Over 11,000 steps per day

Once you have a more accurate idea of your activity level, you can make it a goal to gradually increase your step count. If you're taking fewer than 7,500 steps per day, you could set a goal to increase your step count every week by 1,000 steps per day, until you get into the "Active"

## CALL NEAT "EXERCISE"

Walking around the house doing housework, or having a physical job is technically a source of NEAT, but if you think of it as exercise, you may actually get even more benefit, according to research by the Stanford psychologist Alia Crum.[20] In her study, a group of housekeepers working in hotels were told that their jobs counted as exercise and met the criteria for an active lifestyle. A control group was not told this. The group that was told their jobs counted as exercise burned more energy and got fitter than the control group. Think of your NEAT activities as exercise and you may get even more benefit from them.

category. If you're already there, you may want to increase your steps to become "Very Active."

Here are some more simple ways to increase your NEAT. All of these will add to your daily step count and fuel usage, sometimes significantly:

- **MOVE MORE AT HOME.** Cook meals from scratch, clean more vigorously, do yard work. There is always a lot to be done at home that you might not be doing because you're "busy" sitting and looking at a screen. Get up and get those things done.

- **REDUCE YOUR SCREEN TIME.** Set limits for television and computer time. You could require yourself to get your steps in before turning on the TV.

- **MOVE DURING YOUR MEDIA TIME.** Get up and walk around, fold laundry, do sit-ups and push-ups, or work out while watching TV or listening to podcasts. Jog in place during commercials—it might look ridiculous but it can really help you get your steps in.

- **WALK MORE.** Walking is easy, so you can multitask. Walk around when you're on the phone (this is what Bluetooth headphones are for). Walk to do errands rather than drive, when possible.

- **MOVE ON YOUR BREAKS.** Between classes, on coffee breaks, or whenever you need to stand up and stretch, get up and walk around instead of sitting and scrolling or checking your email. I've learned how to check my email while walking.

- **GET UP EARLIER.** Studies show that people in midlife who get up earlier tend to walk twenty to thirty more minutes than people who stay up later and sleep in.[21]

- **BE INEFFICIENT.** Bring your grocery bags in one at a time. Take things up- or downstairs to put them away one at a time.

- **MOVE AFTER MEALS.** Make a habit of walking for fifteen minutes after every meal.

- **MOVE FOR CREATIVITY.** Walk around while brainstorming or thinking through a problem—research shows that walkers are 81 to 100 percent more creative than sitters.[22]

- **SOCIALIZE ON THE GO.** Take a walk with a friend instead of sitting and eating or drinking. Get together with friends for activities like group workouts or outdoor playdates with kids.

- **WALK THE DOG.** People who have dogs tend to get more steps during the day. One study showed that dog owners walked 22 minutes more and took 2,760 more steps each day than people without dogs.[23] Dog owners are also four times more likely to meet the physical activity guidelines of 150 minutes per week.[24]

- **WALK OR RIDE YOUR BIKE TO WORK OR THE GYM,** if you can.

- **EMPLOY THE THREE-FOR-THIRTY RULE.** Set your smartwatch or phone to remind you to move for three minutes every thirty minutes while working.

- **TAKE THE STAIRS** whenever you can.

- **PARK FAR AWAY FROM THE ENTRANCE.** Even at the grocery store, park at the back of the parking lot.

## BETTER WORKSTATIONS, MORE NEAT

If you are a knowledge worker or otherwise sit at a desk all day, there are ways to change your workstation to encourage movement[25] as well as increase productivity. Here are three ideas you might consider:

- **UNDER-DESK ELLIPTICAL DEVICES** allow you to pedal while you sit.

- **STANDING DESKS.** I build these wherever I go. You can make a standing desk with just a piece of plywood and two stacks of books. You don't have to go out and buy one, although if you want to, there are some nice ones that adjust to many different heights so you can change the height and sit back down when you need to with just a small adjustment. Research[26] suggests that using sit-stand workstations reduces waist circumference and may also improve perceived workload, discomfort, and psychological strain from work.

- **TREADMILL DESKS.** These can help you get more steps in during the day—especially when you're reading and not necessarily writing—though they do tend to be expensive. A systematic review of standing and treadmill desks in the workplace showed that people who used them had reduced waist circumference, lower LDL, and increased HDL.[27]

- **MOVE AT YOUR DESK.** Swivel your chair, twist your torso, stretch your arms. Get up and jump up and down, and do some squats, wall sits, and planks.

## Postural Alignment

Movement isn't just about walking around during the day. It's also about something as subtle as how you sit and how you stand. You can sit and stand actively or passively, and this is largely a matter of posture.

Good posture can increase how much energy you burn. It can also prevent you from getting injured and can relieve chronic pain that could keep you from moving around. Unfortunately, we've largely lost the tradition of teaching kinesthetic awareness. People used to show children how to hold up their own bodies by physically moving them into the right positions, and posture used to be taught in grade school. Now we have devices to prop babies up and we don't pay much attention to how children are sitting or walking because this is no longer an expectation in our culture. Generations have now grown up into adults with bad posture. If you compare a human spine from 1911 to a spine from 1990, the modern spine has a much more exaggerated curvature. Author Esther Gokhale, LAc, who is somewhat famous in Silicon Valley for being the back pain expert to all the tech geniuses who spend a ton of time in front of screens, writes that "the biggest risk factor for back pain, as yet unidentified and underappreciated, is posture."[28]

The consequences of poor posture include a weakened pelvic floor, which can lead to problems for women with age, including organ prolapse and urinary incontinence.[29] As the human pelvis has become more retroverted, the pubic bone, which should be supporting the pelvic organs, is moved out from being directly under the organs to the back, and this puts a strain on the pelvic floor. This can cause sexual dysfunction in both women and men, and decreasing sexual arousal and frequency of orgasms in women, as well as weak ejaculation in men. Sitting and standing up straight can literally improve your sex life.

Over time, poor posture can lead to disc narrowing, a common problem in people who bend over a lot in their work. It can also lead to shoulder impingement and pain, tension headaches, fatigue, and pain down through the joints, from hip to knee to foot. Poor posture may also create the groundwork for thoracic outlet syndrome, a group of disorders related to compression of blood vessels or nerves between the collarbone and first rib, or the nerve roots of the neck vertebrae. This can happen when people sit or stand with their head forward, like toward a computer screen or a phone, and hips tilted back, leading to tightening of the hip flexors and shortening of the hip extensors. This jutting out of the neck compresses the muscles and nerves. Symptoms include upper limb pain, numbness, tingling, and weakness that get worse with shoulder and neck movement.[30] You can also develop temporomandibular joint dysfunction (TMJ) from bad posture because of the tension it causes in the muscles of the neck and jaw. The cascade of effects from poor posture can really influence every part of your body. In many ways, posture makes all other movement possible—or impossible.

I have found the most profound improvements in posture have come from working consistently with bodyworkers or Rolfing therapists. These modalities are different than typical massage. Bodywork involves not just receiving a deep tissue massage but also developing a mental relationship with your body. The therapist enables you to connect the tension stored in your body with your life experiences. Often with tension release, there is emotional release that you can tie to specific memories, almost as though they were stored in your body before being let go. Rolfing is a fairly painful (and endorphin-inducing) form of deep tissue manipulation that involves moving your fascia (connective tissue) back into proper alignment so that your body can support itself more effectively. I recommend these modalities to my patients because for me personally, they have led to breakthroughs in my relationship to myself and resulted in better posture. There is also a good deal of scientific literature to back their efficacy.

Good posture also has psychological benefits: how you carry your body affects the way you think and feel about yourself. There is a bidirectional relationship between how we move and how we feel, and you can change how you feel by changing how you move. Posture can establish social dominance and increase feelings of power, especially with the adoption of power poses, like standing with hands on your hips, keeping legs spread apart, and leaning back with confidence.[31] I employ a power pose on Zoom calls, sitting with my hands up behind my head and my elbows stretched out. It makes me feel strong, especially when I'm on calls with men more powerful than I am.

As you work on your posture, you will notice that you start to feel better, and from there, it becomes a self-reinforcing cycle. Once your body realigns and your muscles and joints get used to the "new" position of standing on your skeleton, you'll realize that it takes more energy and work to maintain and compensate for poor posture—hanging your muscles off your body—than it does to have correct posture. By not standing up straight and not sitting properly, you drain away energy. Proper posture promotes energy efficiency.

Technology often compromises people's posture when sitting because we all look down at our phones. This impairs postural balance, both in older and in younger people.[32] The farther forward you hold your head, the more weight your neck must bear. If your head is straight over your neck, you are holding ten to twelve pounds. With just a fifteen-degree forward bend, that load becomes twenty-seven pounds. At thirty degrees, it's forty pounds. At forty-five degrees, it's forty-nine pounds, and a sixty-degree forward tilt is equivalent to a sixty-pound load on your neck.[33]

Recently I started holding my phone up in front of me at eye level. It looks a little crazy but nobody cares because everybody else is busy looking at their own phone. All that looking down puts a lot of pressure on your neck, so avoid doing this as much as possible.

### POSTURE AND BLOOD OXYGEN

When you don't sit up straight, you compress your lungs, so you don't breathe as deeply, and you don't get as much oxygen to your brain. This is something you can track. Many smartwatches and other trackers have a blood oxygen tracker. These show you how much oxygen you're getting throughout the day. Ideally, you should be at 100 percent, but this can go down due to bad posture, stress, or just shallow breathing (which can happen when you're stressed or sometimes when you're just checking email). If you start tracking and notice your blood oxygen is regularly lower than 99–100 percent, experiment to see if changing your posture raises your number.

## How to Sit and Stand

Achieving consistent good posture isn't just about suddenly standing up straight or sitting up straight. It can involve unlearning years of habits that are ingrained in your muscles. You may have to retrain your body. It's kind of like learning a new athletic skill, but the effort is worth it.

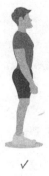 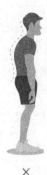

✓                    ✗

Once you learn better posture, it becomes easier and your body starts to accommodate properly.

If you look at the illustration above, you can see how, when you slump, your muscles support your bones, but when you stand up straight, your bones support your muscles.

Posture is important when both standing and sitting. When sitting, think of your body as existing on a set of parallel and perpendicular planes in space.[34] Pay particular attention to these aspects of your sitting posture:

1. *Hold your chin parallel to the ground.*

2. *Be sure both shoulders, both hips, and both knees are at the same height. For example, don't hold one shoulder higher or sit with one knee hiked up.*

3. *Point your knees and feet forward.*

4. *Look straight ahead. Your eyes should be level with the center of your screen. If they aren't, adjust either the height of your screen or the height of your seat.*

5. *Your torso and thighs should be at a ninety-degree angle, hinged at the hip, when you sit.*

6. *Your upper and lower arms should also be at ninety degrees when you are using your keyboard or writing. If they aren't, adjust your chair or desk.*

7. *Avoid slumping and holding your body in curves. Think in terms of nice right angles.*

8. *Even if you use a standing desk, you can maintain these planes. Especially be sure your desk allows you to type with your arms at a right angle and your eyes looking at the middle of the screen.*

When standing, it's also important to avoid curved shapes, to keep your skeleton aligned. Here is how to use postural alignment therapy, or PAT (a system originally developed by anatomical physiologist Pete Egoscue[35]), to stand correctly.[36] The goal here is to get your shoulders over your hips, your hips over your knees, and your knees over your ankles. When standing:

1. *Brace your stomach muscles as if someone were about to punch you, or like you are moving between two people trying not to touch them. This activates your core.*

2. *Stand with your feet two fists-width apart—be sure you can fit two fists between your feet, at both the toes and the heels.*

3. *Move around a bit until you feel your body settling in the center, evenly distributed over your full foot, not just on the balls or the heels. If you can lift up your toes or your heels without shifting, you aren't balanced yet.*

4. *Lift your shoulders up, then move them back and down, as if you were putting your shoulder blades in your back pockets. (This is a small movement, in the direction of your pockets.)*

5. *Imagine there is a string attached to the crown of your head, pulling you straight up. This will help center your head over your skeleton. Your head should not stick forward and your chin should be parallel to the ground. People often have to consciously pull their head straight back to get it over the shoulders.*

6. *Soften your knees. Don't lock them. They should feel neutral, not stuck in place, not bent forward, and not hyperextending backward. Look in a mirror to check.*

7. *Ask yourself: Am I on my skeleton? (Good.) Or am I hanging on my muscles? (Bad.)*

8. *Stay here for a few minutes, noticing how it feels to stand correctly. Everything is connected and the ground supports you. Your weight is evenly distributed.*

9. *Check this several times a day until it becomes a habit.*

## Just Play

Play is a way to move that prepares you for the unexpected because it isn't built on rote motions you do over and over. It's about moving in surprising and different ways, like kids do. This can keep you more mobile, more flexible, and safer. Imagine you suddenly have to run to catch a bus and you step on an uneven piece of pavement. You could sprain your ankle and go down, or you could train your body to expect the unexpected, keeping you from falling because you are used to walking on uneven surfaces in your play training.

Play could involve those things kids do, like hopscotch, cartwheels, rolling down a hill, and playing tag, or you can design your own way to do it. Go at your own pace, and work on making the transitions from one movement to the next graceful and smooth. Don't worry about how you're supposed to do it or how it looks.[37] Play isn't competitive. It's about natural movement. There are ten groups of natural movements you can dip into when you play:

1. WALKING, *in different places, on different surfaces, and in different directions*
2. RUNNING, *fast, slow, in a straight line, in a crooked line*
3. JUMPING, *like jumping rope or jumping over things*
4. QUADRUPEDAL MOVEMENT, *which is crawling on hands and knees, bear crawling, or rolling forward or backward*
5. CLIMBING, *which could be climbing a tree, climbing a rope, climbing rocks*
6. EQUILIBRIUM (BALANCE), *like standing on one foot, or playing on a slack line or a balance beam*
7. THROWING *rocks into a lake, throwing a ball, throwing a stick for a dog*
8. LIFTING *heavy things—kids, packages, shopping bags*
9. SWIMMING, *in a pool or in a natural body of water*

10. **DEFENDING**, *which can be play fighting or, if worse comes to worst, real fighting*

I suggest working some play into every day. You can do it for a few minutes or longer, but it's a serious (and fun) way to increase your body's physical adaptability and stay more mobile.

While incorporating NEAT, steps, posture work, and play into your life can drive big changes in your metabolic and mitochondrial health, getting enough exercise is also important. NEAT and good posture won't give you the cardiorespiratory, strength, flexibility, or even mental health gains you can get with true exercise. You can take your physiological resilience farther with a purposeful, systematic, and intelligent approach to working out. Read on to learn more about how you can biohack your physical fitness through more structured exercise.

---

### EVERYDAY MOVEMENT BIOHACKS IN THIS CHAPTER

- Take every opportunity you can to move.

- Use an accelerometer to get an idea of how much you move during the day to gauge your baseline and see if you can get your steps above seven thousand per day.

- When cleaning or doing housework or yard work, see yourself as doing exercise to get enhanced benefits.

- Revamp your workstation with a standing or treadmill desk and make sure to use good ergonomics.

- Stand up and move around every thirty minutes during the day.

- Train your standing posture.

- Train your sitting posture.

- Track your blood oxygen percentage and notice when your posture is affecting your oxygen uptake.

- Do some play training. Try all ten types of movement.

# CHAPTER 5

# Biohacking Energy Through Exercise

Lack of activity destroys the good condition of every human being, while movement and methodical physical exercise save it and preserve it.

—Plato

Exercise benefits every facet of physical health. It reduces stress, creates stronger muscles and bones, enhances mobility, and increases energy.[1] Regular exercise has also been shown to offer a host of nonphysical side effects, too, from improved mood to better social relationships, self-confidence, and emotional control. Even just walking and stretching can significantly improve quality of life in older people, and research consistently bears out that any amount of exercise improves quality of life as compared to not exercising at all.[2] As one study concluded, even as adults, "we should still have recess."[3]

I've been on a long journey with fitness. I was a competitive runner in high school, but once I hit my twenties, all I did was sit in my chair and study. Aside from yoga in medical school, I was mostly sedentary throughout my twenties, and my ability to focus steadily worsened. By the time I got to my residency, I had destroyed my energy level through lack of movement. I got hit with a viral infection and found myself chronically fatigued.

It wasn't until I was in my late thirties that I discovered a theory known as the adaptive capacity model (ACM),[4] which suggests that if you don't use your body or your mind, your body will produce less energy and fewer brain connections because it has not been "asked" to make more. (It's no coincidence that this is how the mitochondria work.) When we exercise and use our brains, the body anticipates our increased needs for tomorrow. By not exercising in my twenties, I was degrading my energy levels and my brain function. I was given a prescription for Adderall so that I could focus, but taking a pill didn't fix anything. The root cause of my dysfunction was energy deficiency.

It took me ten years to rebuild my fitness—about as long as it took me to lose it. This was a gradual process. I started going to the YMCA and stretching, going to Feldenkrais classes, and using the sauna. I started walking to work instead of driving. Slowly I began adding kettlebells (using apps to give me workouts with them) and eventually bought power blocks (a type of stackable dumbbell) and started using online workout programs. I learned how to use a gym and ran to farmers markets and around parks. I began to see myself as an athlete again. It took me slow, steady progress to get to the point where I now feel confident enough to do any kind of physical activity and welcome the challenge.

If you're new to exercise, start low, go slow, and titrate up. Going too hard too fast is a recipe for injuring yourself. The body prefers slow, steady additions of movement. It's extraordinarily important to realize where you are in your fitness journey and listen to your body's feedback as you increase your exercise.

Exercise is truly a miracle tool, if there ever was one; it offers both immediate and long-lasting benefits, giving you more energy now and compressing morbidity down the line. It's one of the most powerful things you can do for your mind and body, and it might just be the easiest, least expensive, and most effective biohack available to everyone.

Exercise increases mitochondrial output. Your muscles are rich with mitochondria. When you exercise and strengthen them, it's as though you're recharging and building new battery packs. Exercise also boosts the number and function of mitochondria throughout your body, specifically in important organs like your heart, lungs, and brain.

Exercise increases autophagy (cleaning out dead cells) and mitophagy (clearing out damaged mitochondria). This makes room for fresh cells and gets the waste out.[5]

Exercise improves brain function, and it enhances cognition by releasing brain-derived neurotrophic factor (BDNF), a chemical that increases neurogenesis (the production of more neurons), especially when the exercise is high intensity. BDNF allows for the recruitment of mitochondria to your neurons to provide the power supply to build new neural connections.[6] More connections lead to better memory, learning, and mood normalization, and reduced risk of dementia in old age.[7] According to a 2020 study, after just one twenty-minute session of moderate-intensity exercise, blood flow to the hippocampus increases.[8] The hippocampus is associated with memory and cognitive performance, so the greater the blood flow to the hippocampus, the better your brain works.[9] When you don't exercise, your organ systems reduce their capacity, and your brain begins atrophying and aging prematurely, as an energy-saving strategy.[10]

And exercise combats aging. The mitochondrial theory of aging posits that aging is caused by the accumulation of damaged mitochondrial DNA and mitochondria, compromising mitochondrial function and reducing energy capacity.[11] To delay the degeneration so often associated with aging, according to this theory, we need to boost our oxygen-carrying capacity and increase our functional mitochondrial mass. Exercise accomplishes both of these goals quickly and effectively.

In a study testing this theory,[12] researchers created a group of genetically modified mice with a defect that accelerated their aging process. When the mice were subjected to five months of endurance activity, they started making more mitochondria again, and their cells stopped mutating and dying. In another study,[13] researchers created a group of genetically modified mice with a defect that switched off mitochondria production when the mice were given a drug. The result was rapid, with the mice exhibiting visible signs of premature aging, including wrinkled and inflamed skin and hair loss. Then the researchers stopped administering the drug, restoring the mice's mitochondrial production. This had the dramatic effect of aging the mice in reverse. Their skin unwrinkled, their hair grew back, and in a few months, they looked completely normal again.

Hacking mitochondrial health is going to play an important role in future healthcare technologies—companies are already working on supplements and medicines that enhance mitophagy (throwing out the spent batteries/mitochondria that no longer carry a charge). For now, the best intervention for boosting mitochondrial quality control is exercise. If you want to optimize your health, prevent chronic disease, and resist becoming frail with age, exercise.

So just do it, as the saying goes. Everybody knows how to do basic exercises—walking, jogging, sit-ups, push-ups. For every ability level and mobility level, there is something you can do. Try to exercise for about thirty minutes on most days and your mitochondria will step up energy production to match what you're doing. But beyond just doing it, you can do it *better*. Let's get into the details about exercise: how much, how often, how intense, and what to do.

## How Much to Exercise

If you want to live longer, even the minimum amount generally recommended—one hundred fifty minutes a week for adults—can decrease your risk of dying prematurely by 31 percent, compared to those who never exercise.[14] Some people think that's not enough for optimal fitness, and it's probably not. Government guidelines are generally designed for the needs of the majority of the population, not optimization, but if you increase your exercise to an hour a day, statistically you become 39 percent less likely to die early. If you want all the general health benefits of exercise, government physical activity guidelines suggest:

1. *To move throughout the day more and sit less—they note that some physical activity is always better than none.*
2. *For substantial health benefits, adults should do a minimum of 150 minutes (2 hours and 30 minutes) to 300 minutes (5 hours) a week of moderate-intensity, or 75 minutes (1 hour and 15 minutes) to 150 minutes of vigorous-intensity aerobic physical activity, and preferably a combination of different exercise intensities throughout the week.*
3. *For even more health benefits, engage in muscle-strengthening activities at moderate or greater intensity using all major muscle groups on 2 or more days a week.*[15]

It's hard to get too much moderate exercise. Even at ten or more times the recommended minimum of low-to-moderate-intensity exercise or leisure activities, there is no evidence of harm,[16] although most people don't have the time or inclination to exercise that much. However, it's different when it comes to extreme exercise, which can be harmful if you overdo it, especially for the heart. According to the American Heart Association,[17] exercising too hard if you are unfit or are unused to exercise can increase the risk of a sudden heart attack, especially in people who are susceptible to heart problems (and not everyone knows they are susceptible). Extreme amounts of exercise at very high intensity may also accelerate calcification of the arteries of the heart, fibrosis of the myocardium, and atrial fibrillation. Remember, exercise is a stressor. To be hormetic, the stress must be intermittent, include recovery, and not be too extreme, or it will start to break down the body.

The maximum amount of vigorous exercise you should perform

per week is an hour a day for six days. Exercising vigorously, every day, seven days a week increases your risk of mortality.[18] Taking a day off is imperative for proper recovery from high-intensity exercise. Individuals who are over forty-five years of age probably shouldn't perform more than four to five cumulative hours per week of vigorous exercise. The Million Women Study—the largest women's health study in the world, analyzing the health of over one million women between the ages of fifty and sixty-four[19]—showed that regular physical activity dramatically reduced the risk of heart events in women, but those who didn't take at least one day off from strenuous activity per week lost the cardioprotective effects of exercise.[20] The conclusion of the research is that *no exercise and extreme exercise both pose health risks, but there is no limit to the amount of moderate-intensity exercise you can perform.*[21]

## HOW TO USE RESTING HEART RATE
## TO DETERMINE FITNESS

Your heart rate when you are at rest, such as first thing in the morning, is a primary indicator of cardiovascular fitness and heart health. Measure your resting heart rate using a wearable heart rate tracker or by feeling the pulse on your wrist and counting the beats for fifteen seconds, then multiplying the number by four. Do this several mornings in a row to get an average. To interpret your results, consult the following chart. A lower resting heart rate is usually indicative of higher physical fitness, which is associated with lower rates of heart disease. Higher resting heart rate is associated with lower cardiac fitness and increased risk of heart disease, especially heart rates between 81 and 90, which, according to a 2013 study in *Heart,* doubled the risk of cardiac events[22] (this study was in men, but a resting heart rate this high isn't good for women either and likely indicates a similar risk). Resting heart rates above 90 tripled the risk of death.

# How Intense: Determine Exercise Intensity

The table above can help you properly gauge your exercise intensity, or how hard you exercise:[23]

|  | *Moderate Intensity* | *Vigorous Intensity* |
| --- | --- | --- |
| **HOW IT FEELS** | Somewhat hard | Challenging |
| **YOUR BODY'S RESPONSE** | Your breathing quickens but you're not out of breath. | Your breathing is deep and rapid. |
|  | You develop a light sweat after 10 minutes. | You develop a light sweat after only a few minutes of activity. |
|  | You can carry on a conversation, but you can't sing. | You can't say more than a few words without pausing for a breath. |
| **PERCENTAGE OF MAXIMUM HEART RATE** | 50–70% of your maximum heart rate | 70–85% of your maximum heart rate |
| **EXAMPLES** | Brisk walking | Running |
|  | Biking with light effort, about 10 mph) | Sports |
|  | Yoga, Pilates, Barre | Biking with hard effort (about 14 mph), including a spin class |
|  | Household chores such as vacuuming or mopping | Lifting heavy weights |

You can also determine your intensity by calculating your maximum heart rate, or how high your heart rate should go during exercise. To do this, subtract your age from 220. If you are 30 years old, your maximum heart rate would be 190. If you are 40, it would be 180. I recommend wearables with built-in heart rate monitors that track exercise intensity.

- Let's say you are 35. Your maximum heart rate is 220–35 = 185.

- 50 percent of your maximum heart rate would be 185 x 0.5 = 92.5.

- 70 percent of your maximum heart rate would be 185 x 0.7 = 129.5.

- 85 percent of your maximum heart rate would be 185 x 0.85 = 157.25.

Now let's talk about what kinds of exercise to do and the benefits of different kinds of exercise for different purposes.

## Biohacking Cardio

Cardiovascular exercise is any activity that elevates your heart rate to the point where you are mildly stressing your heart and lungs, and it is the best way to get healthy and fit heart, lungs, and mitochondria. Activities like jogging, running, dancing, cycling, elliptical trainers, treadmills, stair climbers, rowing machines, and kickboxing are effective for creating new, healthy mitochondria. Some people wonder if walking can count as cardio. Maybe. A study published in the journal *Applied Physiology, Nutrition, and Metabolism* found if you walk more than 7,500 steps a day, you can probably meet the recommendations for moderate physical activity. That said, you're going to have to walk at a pretty brisk pace. If you're strolling along, you aren't going to get your heart rate up. If you want the benefits of improved heart health, mood, and longevity, you need to exercise to the point where your heart rate is at least 50 to 70 percent of your maximum heart rate. Getting a heart rate monitor can help you track this while working out.

Cardio training increases cardiorespiratory fitness, which is the capacity of your circulatory and respiratory systems to bring oxygen to the mitochondria in your muscles, so they can make energy you can use during exercise.[24] Cardiorespiratory fitness is one of your most important measures of health. The forty-thousand-person Aerobics Center Longitudinal Study showed that low cardiorespiratory fitness, or CRF, predicted premature death better than any other risk factor.[25] But remember, even having good cardiorespiratory fitness doesn't mean that you're protected from the risks of a sedentary lifestyle. A 2018 study in the *Journals of Gerontology* showed that among older adults, physical inactivity still predicted a higher chance of premature death, completely independent of cardiorespiratory fitness.[26] No matter how fit you are now, you have to keep moving, so don't forget what you learned about NEAT in the previous chapter.

The best way to evaluate your cardiorespiratory fitness is to measure your $VO_2$ max, which is a measure of your aerobic capacity. It's the maximum amount of oxygen your body can burn during high-intensity exertion, expressed in milliliters per kilogram per minute. Here's how to find yours:

- SIMPLE: To get a quick and dirty estimate of your $VO_2$ max, calculate 90 percent of your maximum heart rate, as you calculated above (which, if you were 35, would be 167 beats per minute), or go to WorldFitnessLevel.org and plug in your resting heart rate, maximum heart rate, and waist circumference.

- BETTER: You can get a reasonably good measurement of your $VO_2$ max using certain fitness trackers. Track an outdoor twenty-minute walk, run, or hike on your wearable. Do this a few days in a row to get an average estimate of your $VO_2$ max.

- BEST: To get a really accurate measure of your $VO_2$ max requires a test in a laboratory or clinic while exercising, typically on a treadmill, for twenty minutes. Bring a friend to a $VO_2$ max testing center and have them cheer for you while you are on the treadmill so you run as fast and hard as you can.

The average $VO_2$ max for women is around 30 mL/kg per minute, and about 35 mL/kg per minute for men. Anything above 50 is excellent. Lifelong endurance athletes have the highest $VO_2$ max when compared to sedentary people (for example, Lance Armstrong's was 84). Although $VO_2$ max declines with age, an athlete's lowest level with age will still be higher than a sedentary person's highest level at any point in their life.

If your $VO_2$ max is lower than you hoped, know that you can steadily improve it with regular aerobic exercise. $VO_2$ max is a key predictor of longevity because it's highly linked to functional capacity and human performance, as well as cardiovascular capacity, which keeps your heart ticking. With more movement, you have more batteries and capacitors, and with more capacitors, you have more capacity to live a lot longer.

## HIIT: Cardio in Half the Time

High-intensity interval training, or HIIT, is one of the most efficient ways to improve your cardiorespiratory fitness. The basic principle behind HIIT is to alternate all-out, highest-possible-intensity effort with moderate to low effort, for recovery. There are a lot of ways to do it, and a lot of opinions about the right way to do it, but the basics are to exercise as hard and fast as you can for a short interval (e.g., thirty to sixty seconds), then recover at a slow to moderate pace for another interval (e.g., sixty to ninety seconds). You can get the benefits of a thirty- to forty-five-minute moderate-intensity workout in ten to fifteen minutes.

I like HIIT because you can get the same benefits as cardio in a fraction of the time, and because it's particularly good at improving both the number and function of mitochondria.[27] Additionally, HIIT uses up all the glycogen in your liver quickly, emptying your glycogen "sink" in a similar way to fasting (page 152). HIIT also increases the production of growth hormone, which builds muscle, burns fat, and reverses many of the metabolic signs of aging.

You can turn just about any type of cardio into a HIIT workout: walking, running, swimming, cycling, rowing, calisthenics like burpees and jump squats, weight lifting, jumping rope, or cardio machines at the gym like the elliptical trainer, treadmill, or stationary bike.

Also, less is more. I personally don't do this kind of exercise more than once a week. A 2021 study in *Cell Metabolism* demonstrated that you're better off limiting HIIT to a maximum of 60 to 90 minutes per week, because at 150 minutes per week, you can experience mitochondrial dysfunction and problems maintaining glucose tolerance.[28]

I've included below some beginner-to-intermediate HIIT workouts you can try. A caveat: if you are not engaging in a consistent exercise regimen or are highly stressed, please do not try HIIT without your doctor's clearance.

## Sample HIIT Workouts

*Walking: Repeat 3 times for a 9-minute workout*
- EFFORT INTERVAL: Walk 2 minutes at 90% effort, or 5.0 mph on the treadmill
- RECOVERY INTERVAL: Walk 1 minute at normal effort, or 3 mph on the treadmill

*Running, Cycling, or Swimming: Repeat 8 times in 4 minutes*
- BEYOND MAXIMUM EXERTION: 20 seconds
- RECOVERY INTERVAL: 10 seconds

*Calisthenics: Repeat 2 to 5 times*
- WORK INTERVAL: 10 jump squats + 10 push-ups
- RECOVERY INTERVAL: 30 seconds stretching

*Weight lifting: Repeat 2 to 5 times*
- WORK INTERVAL: 10 back squats + 10 barbell rows
- RECOVERY INTERVAL: 30-second rest

## Strength Training: Building Your Mitochondrial Power Grid

If there is one form of exercise I consider nonnegotiable for optimal health and longevity, it's weight training. Weight training builds bone and muscle, amplifies metabolism, and gives you more overall tone and strength. Your muscles are dense with mitochondria, and these little power plants act like electrical transmission wires, distributing energy throughout the muscle in a gridlike network.[29] If we let our muscles waste as we get older, we're essentially losing our power, which means we won't have the capacity to maintain our physical structure, and that leads to frailty. How you use your muscles now could determine whether you'll be able to stand up from a chair (not to mention the floor) without help decades down the line. It may seem far away, but you can influence your fate now. It's immensely important for women to perform weight-bearing exercise and build their bone and muscle density. Falls can cut a life short in the blink of an eye.

People new to weight training often waste time in a gym because they don't know what to do or how to get the real benefits. It's also easy to injure yourself if you don't have the right form. I recommend that you start out with a trainer or instructor, or at least take a class, to learn how to make gains and progress in strength, balance, and flexibility. A 2017 study[30] of older adults that reviewed multiple studies comparing supervised versus unsupervised training programs found that supervised resistance and/or balance training improved balance and strength/power much better than unsupervised programs. You might not need to keep working with a trainer. A few sessions showing you the ropes might be enough. Learn the basic machines and the basic moves, and get help creating a progressive strength-training program you can work on yourself. Trainers can also provide accountability and help motivate you to show up.

These are some basic moves everyone should know if they are weight training. Some can be done with free weights or bands, and some require machines. Ask your trainer to show you how to do these, or watch a trainer do these online:

- Squat
- Dead lift
- Pull-up
- Seated dumbbell shoulder press
- Leg press
- Bent-over row
- Upright row
- Dip
- Bench press
- Biceps curl
- Triceps push-down
- Seated cable row
- Lat pull-down
- Crunch

Once you know how to do these, choose six exercises and do two to four sets of each exercise with eight to ten repetitions per set and one- to two-minute rest intervals between sets. Mix up the muscle groups to make sure you are allowing recovery in between workouts. On a typical week I'll do a leg day, a back and biceps day, a chest and triceps day, and a full-body day with abs.

You don't need a gym or even weights to strength-train. During the COVID-19 pandemic, I found myself temporarily without a gym, so I started incorporating body-weight workouts at home. These types of routines are great for conditioning because some employ plyometrics (power-producing moves like jumping) and isometrics (holding a muscle in a position that causes fatigue). Here's a sample workout:

- 5 push-ups + 5 squats + 5 sit-ups: 20 rounds
- 10 push-ups + 10 sit-ups + 10 squats: 10 rounds
- 30 seconds each: bear crawl, crab walk, walking lunges, broad jumps, repeated for 12 minutes
- Air squats and push-ups: 12, then 15, then 9
- 3 vertical jumps + 3 squats + 3 long jumps: 5 rounds
- 30 seconds each: plank position, hold bottom of a squat, hollow rock hold: 10 rounds
- 30 seconds on, 30 seconds off: jumping squats (4 minutes), split jumps (4 minutes), tuck jumps (4 minutes)
- 10 vertical jumps + 10 push-ups + 10 sit-ups: 4 rounds
- Handstand, 1 minute + hold bottom of squat, 1 minute: 5 rounds
- 50 air squats: 5 rounds (rest for the same amount of time it took to do 50 reps)

## Protein Considerations for Exercise

There are two parts to building and maintaining muscle: the physical challenge to the muscle, and the time and raw material it takes to build the muscle back after the challenge. That raw material is protein. When you begin any exercise program, monitor your protein intake with a food-tracking app that breaks down macros (protein, carbs, fat).

It took me a while to figure out why protein recommendations were so varied, so I will save you time and simplify it here in this list:

- The recommended daily allowance (RDA) is 0.8 g/kg per day, but this is probably too low if you exercise regularly.

- Patients with diabetes and chronic kidney disease (who are at risk for too much protein putting stress on their kidneys) need a protein intake of 0.8–1 g/kg per day.[31]

- Individuals over 65 need a minimum of 1.2 g/kg per day to maintain proper muscle mass to avoid frailty.

- Malnourished, acute or chronically ill, or injured older people, and anyone who doesn't exercise regularly, should aim for 1.2 to 1.5 g/kg per day.[32]

- General athletes should get 1.4 to 1.7 g/kg per day.

- Runners require 1.4 to 1.7 g/kg per day to meet the needs of their training. But new research suggests endurance athletes may need upwards of 1.8 g/kg per day. The researchers pointed out that male endurance runners often met the recommended intake of 1.8 g/kg per day, but female runners often missed this higher mark.[33]

- Weight lifters who want to maintain their muscle mass need a minimum of 1.6 g/kg per day.[34]

Use an online calculator to convert your weight into kilograms. For example, someone who weighs 150 pounds weighs 68 kilograms, so if they are following the RDA, they would be aiming for approximately 54 grams of protein per day. If this person were a weight lifter trying to put on mass, they would need a minimum of 108 grams of protein. An endurance runner would need at least 122 grams of protein (the bare minimum required for muscle growth). Also, keep in mind you want to calculate your protein needs based on your ideal weight so it may be more or less depending on whether you're trying to gain or lose mass.

---

### KNOW YOUR POST-EXERCISE REFUELING WINDOW

The window to refuel after exercise matters to muscle protein synthesis and is different depending on your age and sex. Premenopausal women need thirty grams of protein post-exercise and have a ninety-minute window to refuel. Postmenopausal women need forty grams of protein post-exercise and have a ninety-minute window to refuel. Men need a minimum of twenty grams of protein after a workout and have a three-to-eighteen-hour window to refuel.

---

As we age, two of the biggest threats to our lives are frailty and obesity, and these can lead to falls and metabolic diseases. After sixty-five, we become less responsive to protein as an anabolic stimulus for muscle growth, so when we eat the same amount of protein as when we were younger, we are less able to use it to build muscle. The end result is our muscles waste, so I recommend at least 1.2 g/kg per day of protein if you are over sixty-five. For those who exercise, research suggests the elderly may need forty grams of protein ninety minutes post-exercise to get the most muscle protein synthesis.[35]

Muscle protein synthesis is dependent on having enough amino acids in circulation to provide growth after exercise. Women in particular need enough of the amino acid leucine after exercise. When leucine enters the brain, it sends a signal to the body to make muscles grow. Think of this signal as a cellular switch for growing muscle that gets turned on after you eat enough post-exercise protein. Refueling with leucine-rich foods like Greek yogurt or protein shakes can help.

If you undereat protein, you won't see improvements in your strength or physique, and you'll get extra sore after gym sessions. In a perfect world, we would get all our protein from whole foods, but sometimes it's tough to meet our requirements this way. On days when I don't meet my protein requirements due to work, travel, or general busy-ness, I supplement with 5 grams of essential amino acids (EAAs) to get the muscle protein synthesis signal activated. EAAs are the amino acids that your body can't make on its own, so you must get them from your diet.

If muscle gain is your priority, you might consider protein supplements. A 2020 study[36] showed that dietary protein supplementation

## TOO MUCH PROTEIN?

Scientists who study aging believe that too much protein could accelerate age-related diseases, especially in the context of inadequate exercise. My personal interpretation is that your body uses protein to grow—it's like fertilizer in the garden—and it will increase the growth of whatever you are growing, whether that's muscle or cancer cells. Exercise produces signaling molecules known as myokines, and these send signals to our immune cells to attack and kill cancer cells. Without exercise, we aren't getting these signals, so the growth signals from protein may contribute to weight gain and cancer growth as we age.

Evidence-based nutritional researchers, like Alan Aragon, firmly believe that low protein is a significant threat to longevity because it compromises fat loss, muscle preservation, muscle quality, exercise performance, and cardiometabolic health. Furthermore, a recent review concluded that in humans, BCAA (branched chain amino acid) levels decline with age and are reduced even further with frailty.[37]

I recommend my patients aim for 1.6 g/kg in body weight of protein per day. I like to exercise five days a week, but on rest days or if I am traveling, I occasionally employ protein cycling, which involves limiting protein intake to less than 20 grams a day once a week. This practice of intermittent nutrient deprivation may boost cellular autophagy when you are not exercising.

significantly enhanced muscle strength and size in healthy adults, although this maxes out at about 1.6 g/kg per day. I use both nose-to-tail protein blends (containing hydrolyzed beef, freeze-dried organ meats, bone, and blood) as well as plant-based protein powders. My favorite plant-based protein is made from pea protein, pumpkin seed protein, chia seed protein, coconut protein, and hemp seed protein.

Collagen protein is particularly useful for its glycine content, which shows up as a common deficiency on urine organic acid testing in my practice, in patients who mainly consume muscle meat. Glycine comes from connective tissue like bones and tendons. Glycine has been shown to increase collagen synthesis, and glycine deficiency may contribute to the development of osteoarthritis.[38] My favorite animal-based sources of glycine are collagen protein powder, bone broth protein powder, and bone broth. Sesame seeds, pumpkin seeds, soy, spinach, and pistachios are good sources for vegans.

## Mind-Body Fitness

There is more to exercise than just getting your heart rate up and building your muscles. Good balance and flexibility, which are essential for maintaining mobility and preventing falls as you get older, are also important goals. Exercise also benefits our mental health.

When I was in med school, I was so burned out that the only exercises I could do were yoga and tai chi. I couldn't believe how good I felt after doing these activities. It was the easiest exercise I'd ever done, physically, but it made me feel so positive. Embodied cognition theory explains this effect.[39] According to this theory, the way that we move and manipulate the shape of our bodies, as well as the facial expressions and gestures we make, alter mood and cognitive behavior. It's a bidirectional relationship—the way that we stand, carry ourselves, and move influences how we feel, just like how we feel influences how we move.

This is probably why, for example, dancing makes people feel better and sitting in a slumped position makes people feel worse.

Certain exercises can build more energy into the body, even though they are typically low-energy, low-impact exercises that don't increase heart rate. A study analyzing meditative movement in terms of the unification of Eastern and Western exercise theory[40] demonstrated that practicing qi gong resulted in a state of deep relaxation; balanced muscle tone; improved flexibility and proprioception (feeling where your body is in space); better brain plasticity, coordination, circulation, and balance (related to fall prevention); and increased parasympathetic activity (that "rest and digest" nervous system mode).

The cool thing about mind-body exercises like yoga, tai chi, and qi gong is that they can improve your flexibility, strength, balance, circulation, stimulation of the endocrine glands, and coordination while also inducing the relaxation response. Because qi gong and tai chi use meditative movements that involve focused awareness on the body with explicit attention to breathing, they slow breathing and improve that parasympathetic tone. This is what induces a state of deep relaxation, which balances the autonomic nervous system.

Also, when we perform multiplanar movements, the body behaves in an integrated manner, which improves cognitive function, brain plasticity, neuromuscular coordination, attention, and postural control. Some research even shows that these kinds of meditative movements reduce inflammation, increase immune support, and stimulate DNA repair.[41]

Yoga is a little different from tai chi and qi gong. It's especially good at stimulating the endocrine glands through bends and twists, improving posture and balance, and increasing flexibility and strength, but one of its most interesting benefits might be that it can change how you feel. In 1890, William James posited[42] the theory that although emotions can lead to postures and body states, postures and body states can also lead to (or intensify) emotions. He proposed that we don't just laugh because we're happy—we become happy when we laugh. Yoga facilitates this bidirectional relationship between thoughts/emotions and physical behavior.

As a result, yoga is one of the best activities you can do to cultivate balance—emotional as well as physical. Physically, balance is extremely important for healthspan, and yoga teaches you multiple types of balance:

- STEADY-STATE BALANCE, which is maintaining a sturdy position while you aren't moving (like in mountain pose).

- DYNAMIC STEADY-STATE BALANCE, which is maintaining a steady position while moving through different postures or through space, such as heel to toe in a straight line.

- PROACTIVE BALANCE, which is the anticipation of a predicted postural disturbance (the transitions between yoga poses helps with this).

- REACTIVE BALANCE, which is how you compensate for unpredicted postural disturbance—your functional reflexes, like catching yourself when you're about to fall.[43]

Another interesting thing about yoga is how it can be explained through the scientific lens of piezoelectricity.[44] Piezoelectricity is generated when you bend, stretch, and twist. This creates a kind of stress on the body that is converted into electrical current. Bones and muscles are to some degree spongy and compressible, and they can compress and expand based on what we do with our bodies; this may be part of why exercise that doesn't seem difficult actually gives us more energy. Mechanical stress, pressure, and latent heat create a charge that accumulates in our collagen, tendons, and bones.[45]

There are many types of yoga, including rigorous, strength-based forms like Ashtanga that build lean muscle and flexibility, and gentler forms like yin yoga, which is great for fascia, the connective tissue in the body that surrounds and holds all your organs, blood vessels, muscles, nerves, and bones in place. We carry a lot of tension in our fascia, and there's a theory that we carry emotions and trauma in our fascia, which can harden in response to constant threats. I think of fascia as the fiber-optic cable system of the body. When emotions get stuck, we often experience pain, and a good stretching session can help to process physical and emotional stress.

But as with all exercise, go gently at first. I've seen people get hurt even with yin yoga. If there's something you aren't sure you can do, don't do it, and if anything really hurts, stop. While there's always a little pain if you're stiff, that's stretching pain, not injury pain. Go to a class and learn the poses with an instructor.

## Avoiding Frailty and Maintaining Mobility with Age

Here's a wake-up call: millennials seem to be losing grip strength, which is a basic measure of strength. Women and men under thirty years old have significantly weaker hand grips than people of the same age did in 1985, according to a 2020 study.[46] Losing our grip strength is a frightening harbinger for future frailty in this generation. To avoid frailty, you need to get strong now—not after you have lost your muscle.

Having strong muscles is a major predictor of healthspan and longevity. The inability to walk across a room is what puts most people into a nursing home, and falls are a major cause of disability and death in the elderly. Half of people in their eighties have an increased need for assisted care because of mobility limitations that predispose them to falls, and after a fall and a fracture, 4 percent of elderly people die acutely, 40 percent die within two years, and 60 to 80 percent never regain full function.[47] Falls are a huge issue, especially for people with osteoporosis.

In addition to the physical risk, weak upper and lower body fitness is linked to both depression and anxiety in women in midlife, according to a study published in *Menopause* of more than 1,100 women between the ages of forty-five and sixty-nine.[48] One measure of weakness was handgrip strength, and another was needing a long time to stand up from a chair. Both were associated with increased depression and anxiety symptoms.

Sarcopenia is a condition often associated with aging characterized by loss of muscle and subsequent increased weakness. It's linked with increased disability, falls, hospitalization, nursing home admission, and death. It's characterized by progressive loss of muscle structure (as measured by loss of muscle mass, increased muscle fat, and reduced grip strength) and function (as measured by reduced gait speed and lowered $VO_2$ max). Primary to this process is mitochondrial dysfunction, but as you already know, exercise can reverse this process by increasing mitochondrial health—both strength training and aerobic exercise counteract sarcopenia, with adequate protein intake.[49]

The average person has about ten years of dependent living at the end of life, but those who remain physically active can compress this to an average of one to three years. As a woman, by the time you are twenty-five to thirty, your muscle mass starts decreasing by about 1 percent each year.[50] By seventy, you've lost potentially up to 30 percent of the cross-sectional area of your muscle, and by eighty, it's 40 percent.[51] You'll also lose flexibility and increase rigidity with age, which decreases your range of movement, making it hard to do many activities of daily living.

Bones lose density with age, making them more brittle and prone to fractures and breaks. Women build most of their bone mass as adolescents,[52] and our bones are at their densest at about eighteen years old. After menopause, when estrogen declines, bone density plummets, which can lead to osteoporosis. If we don't reach optimal bone mass during adulthood, we can end up frail and fragile. Lifting weights (and putting any kind of stress on bones) is one of the most effective ways to reclaim some of that bone density as you age. However, research suggests this may be dependent on whether or not you are using estrogen replacement therapy.[53]

It's never too early to work on this. If you really want to achieve physiological resilience, avoid frailty, maintain your mobility as you age, and maintain your aerobic fitness to make more and healthier mitochondria, prioritize fitness: maintain muscle mass and strength with regular resistance exercise, maintain balance and flexibility with exercises that challenge these and improve proprioception, and maintain resilience by moving in unexpected ways. Teach your body to adapt constantly to different training regimens and tackle weakness systematically (such as after an injury).

When you first start exercising, you might not feel great. In fact, you might feel tired, sore, and worn out. But pushing through the first few weeks of pain is so worth it! You won't always have the willpower to get up and get moving, but push through those first few weeks, because exercise will start to feel great and you'll miss it if you skip a few days. Focus on how you will feel after your workout rather than how hard the workout will be. Find exercise you enjoy and find friends to work out with. Join a gym or sign up for classes that are convenient to where you live. Go at your own pace, and remember that it's always better to exercise a little than not at all. It's self-care that will pay off now as well as later, with extended healthspan, energy, strength, mobility, and longevity.

### EXERCISE HACKS IN THIS CHAPTER

- Track your resting heart rate to determine your fitness level.

- Calculate your moderate and vigorous intensity ranges.

- Track your $VO_2$ max to determine your cardiorespiratory fitness.

- Try some sample HIIT workouts.

- Learn basic weight-training exercises.

- Try a bodyweight workout if you can't get to the gym.

- Calculate your personal protein needs based on your activity level.

- Know your protein refueling window.

- Integrate mind-body fitness workouts.

- Plan for reducing frailty risk as you age.

# PART III

# CHARGING YOUR BATTERIES

# CHAPTER 6

# Transforming Food into Energy

Fake food—I mean those patented substances chemically flavored and me-chanically bulked out to kill the appetite and deceive the gut—is unnatural, almost immoral, a bane to good eating and good cooking.

—Julia Child

One of the fundamentals of life is finding fuel to power our bodies. Our mitochondria transform the food we eat into the energy we use. For most of human history, survival meant spending most of our time hunting or gathering food in order to stay alive. It's no wonder food feels, on an instinctual level, so important. And it *is* important. Now, however, the foods available to us have changed dramatically, and our quest for sustenance can become either a health hazard or an opportunity for optimization. The foods you choose can degrade your body and promote chronic disease, or they can make you stronger, healthier, and more resilient.

When it comes to food, there may be plenty of instinctual drives, but I believe most people are legitimately confused about what to eat. People know whole foods are more nutritious than junk food, certainly, but eating is rarely that straightforward. Our food choices are bound up in external cues, like exposure to advertising and tempting smells and tastes, as well as internal cues, like emotions, guilt, indulgence, and not fully understanding the connection between how we eat and how we feel. More than any other question, people continue to ask me: "Dr. Molly, what should I eat?"

The complicated thing about nutrition is that while there are some universal truths, it's also individual. Some foods work really well for some people and really poorly for others. To figure out what works well for you, you're going to have to do some experimenting. It's important to understand that just because an expert says something is "good for you," that doesn't mean it's good for *you*.

Most nutritionists agree on the basics—a healthy diet primarily consists of fiber-rich, plant-based foods such as vegetables, fruit, nuts and seeds, legumes, and whole grains (if you tolerate grain), along with healthy protein like seafood, with low to moderate alcohol consumption. This dietary pattern *generally* supports blood sugar control and a healthy microbiome, although that doesn't tell you anything about what it will do for you personally.

But most people don't eat this way. Instead, the standard American diet is heavy on refined grains, red and processed meats, sugar-sweetened beverages, industrial seed oils, and excessive alcohol consumption (more than about a four-ounce glass of wine a day for women). We know this diet decreases glycemic control, increases diabetes risk, and can lead to digestive disorders and a leaky gut.[1]

The real truth is that this "good and bad" picture has a lot of exceptions. For example, some people (but not everyone) struggle to digest beans and grains, and some people (but not everyone) thrive on red meat. Modern nutrition just isn't one-size-fits-all. Different people will thrive on different foods, and it can take time to figure out what works for your body.

That being said, there are some rules that apply to everyone. In comparison to the first half of the 1900s, we are now consuming far more refined grains, refined sugars, refined vegetable oils, trans fats, and processed meats coming from confined animal operations. If you first focus on eliminating ultra-processed foods (junk food, fast food, and packaged food), you can dramatically improve your health. These foods cause gut dysfunction, inflammation, and disease. If you really want to eat for maximum healthspan, the first step to a healthy diet is eating whole, real food. So check that off your list before worrying about going to the next level.

## Your Guide to Eating Carbohydrates

Carbohydrates are a macronutrient found in foods from vegetables to pastries, so you can't really categorize all carbohydrate-rich foods together. Carbohydrates are important for their fiber and resistant starch, which improve microbiome health, but not every food that is high in carbs has fiber or resistant starch, so if you want to get those, you have to choose wisely. Carbs are in vegetables, and carbs are in candy. You already know that vegetables are good, so let's focus on some things you might not know.

It's important to understand how detrimental to your health added sugars and refined grains really are. Sugar is inflammatory. It raises blood sugar too quickly and can upset microbiome balance, causing overgrowth of more pathogenic, inflammatory bacteria and yeast. The American Heart Association and WHO recommend less than 5 percent of your calories come from added sugar, which is less than twenty-five grams of sugar, or six teaspoons. If you're a pro, you'll aim for less than one teaspoon a day.

Avoiding extra sugar as much as possible is one of the simplest ways that you can reduce blood sugar spikes. Blood sugar spikes, as you'll learn later, can cause blood vessel damage and diabetes. This is why it's so important to know, through tracking, when blood sugar is not under control, and how to manage it to get it back under control. (You'll learn more about how to track and manage blood sugar in chapter 7.)

I recommend avoiding white sugar, brown sugar, agave (which is pure fructose and hard on the liver), concentrated fruit juice, and corn syrup. In small amounts you can eat dates, honey, maple syrup, or a little bit of xylitol and still keep your blood sugar stable. Xylitol may or may not increase intestinal permeability, but it's probably okay here and there (I still wouldn't recommend more than a teaspoon daily). Xylitol is often in gum, which is good for your oral health. I do a little bit of raw honey, which does have some minerals and antioxidants, but it's still sugar, so it's important to be mindful of portions.

### WHAT ABOUT FRUIT SUGAR?

Of all the varieties of sugar (sucrose, dextrose, glucose, fructose), fructose (fruit sugar) is particularly problematic because it goes straight to the liver without being processed through the bloodstream. This is one of the reasons why high-fructose corn syrup is so dangerous. Fructose is more likely to increase visceral fat formation than any other kind of sugar. But that doesn't mean you shouldn't eat fruit. Fruit is good for you, full of vitamins, minerals, phytonutrients, and fiber, and there is zero evidence that fruit causes diabetes. In fact, it's clear that eating whole fruit can protect against diabetes and hypertension, according to a 2021 study[2] (fruit juice has the opposite effect according to some studies—fruit juice doesn't contain the fiber).

But I do think it's good to know how fruit affects your blood sugar, which you can determine by using a continuous glucose monitor or testing your blood sugar an hour after eating fruit (chapter 7). Personally, I avoid the super-high-glycemic fruits like mangoes and pineapples because every time I eat those, I get a blood sugar spike. What's more important to avoid than fruit is excess fructose from juice and soda. Fruit is always a better choice than something with added fructose.

Replacing sugar with a noncaloric sweetener isn't much better and might even be worse. Noncaloric sweeteners like aspartame, sucralose, acesulfame-K, and saccharin have been shown to cause weight gain, impaired glucose metabolism, and cancer in animal studies. Even supposedly healthy sweeteners like mannitol and erythritol can cause GI upset and might increase intestinal permeability.[3] A small amount of monk fruit (which is erythritol) is probably your best bet in this category. Stevia is another good alternative. But no fake sugar should be a big part of your diet. I've definitely seen overconsumption of non-caloric sweeteners contributing to gut dysfunction, dysbiosis, and small intestinal bacterial overgrowth.

Grains are also carbs, and refined grain might as well be sugar for how it affects blood sugar and the microbiome. I don't think it's great to eat a lot of grain of any kind, but if you really want to optimize metabolic health, it's particularly important to avoid white flour, white rice, white pasta, instant oatmeal, and refined corn and potato products (like chips). If you are a serious endurance athlete or extremely good at using glucose (as many serious endurance athletes are, as well as other people who are naturally skinny, have low visceral fat, have fast metabolisms, and struggle to gain weight), you can probably get away with more refined carbohydrates than the average person. But most people who put on a glucose monitor (page 129) will see that these foods cause blood sugar spikes.

Sugar and refined carbs taste really good. They may feel addictive to you. But nobody is making you eat them. If you really want to get the most out of your carbs, they should mainly come from vegetables, fruit, and intact whole grains that aren't ground into flour.

## Your Guide to Fat

Fat is at least as complicated as carbs, and like carbs, some types of fat can harm health and some types are good for health. Here's a brief ranking:

THE WORST: Trans fats, or trans fatty acids, have no redeeming qualities. There is definitive evidence that artificial trans fats—created when liquid vegetable oils get hydrogenated into solid fats—contribute to heart disease.[4] The evidence is so overwhelming that the government has required food companies to phase out trans fats.[5] If you want to

## SORRY, BUT OAT MILK ISN'T A HEALTH FOOD

Oat milk has become the new plant milk of choice, and people think it's good for them, or an improvement over dairy milk. But oat milk is made from grain that has been enzymatically broken down into individual starch molecules. It can spike your blood sugar because it contains maltose, which has an extremely high glycemic index (a measure of the average of how much a food spikes blood sugar), and twelve ounces of oat milk (the amount in a medium latte) has about the same blood sugar impact as a twelve-ounce can of cola.[6] Plus, it often contains industrialized seed oils (the same amount found in a serving of fries). If you need milk, I recommend unsweetened almond, hemp, coconut, or macadamia nut milk.

make sure you aren't consuming them, avoid baked goods made with vegetable shortening (muffins, pies, pastries, and cakes), microwaved popcorn, margarine, and fried fast food (e.g., chicken fingers and fries).

ALSO PROBLEMATIC: If there is one kind of fat you want to examine your intake around, it's vegetable oil. I don't believe on its own that it's necessarily poisonous or as problematic for health as many people claim, but I think it's important to look at the potentially negative health effects of excessive intake of vegetable oil, and the consumption of rancid vegetable oil (which could happen during extraction, storage, and repeated frying).

Today, vegetable oil is a highly refined, industrially processed food product. A hundred years ago, vegetable oil made up a tiny portion of the American diet. We are now consuming significantly more calories from industrially produced vegetable oils, especially soybean, canola, cottonseed, and corn oil, and this has resulted in people now consuming over five hundred calories—about 20 percent of their calories—from vegetable oil every day.[7] That's a lot. Globally, more vegetable oil is produced than poultry, beef, cheese, and butter combined. It's the most consumed food in the world after rice and wheat.

Furthermore, because so much vegetable oil that is consumed has gone rancid due to factory processing, poor shelf stability, or oxidation with repeated frying, it's even more damaging to health. Fried food is delicious, but it is one of the worst things we can consume. The negative effects on health, it is believed, are largely due to consuming heated vegetable oil in the context of fast food and processed snack foods like chips. We know these foods aren't healthy. Are vegetable oils like canola oil on their own toxic to health? Probably not. But consuming vegetable oils in excess, eating fried foods, and binging on ultra-processed snack foods and fast foods certainly is.

## FRUIT OIL INSTEAD OF VEGETABLE OIL

Instead of vegetable oils, I recommend cooking with fruit oils like olive and avocado oils. I do use some coconut oil, duck fat, beef tallow, and lard as well—though I use these sparingly (as I do all oils)—but fruit oils are ideal because they have much lower percentages of omega-6 polyunsaturated fatty acids and more monounsaturated fatty acids, which have a positive impact on cholesterol.[8] In addition, multiple studies have shown that those who consume at least a half tablespoon a day of olive oil in particular have a 14 percent lower risk for cardiovascular disease and an 18 percent lower risk for coronary heart disease[9] than those who don't consume olive oil. Just remember to source your oils from reliable brands, as there are many poor-quality avocado and olive oils on the market.

**BETTER BUT STILL PROBLEMATIC**: Saturated fat is a subject of dietary controversy. Some research says that unsaturated fat is much better for health than saturated fat. Other research says the opposite. The disconnect is in the details.

Saturated fats aren't uniformly bad for health, but we eat too much. Hunters and gathers probably got around 10–15 percent of their calories from saturated fat. In France, the average intake of saturated fat is less than 15 percent of calories. Dietary guidelines in most countries generally recommend less than 10 percent of total calories from saturated fat. Most people in the U.S. consume an average of 21 percent of calories from saturated fat. We should be aiming for between 10 and 15 percent of calories from saturated fat.

Saturated fats on their own are probably not damaging to health, but they are usually eaten with refined carbs. This combination induces a big insulin spike from the carbs along with decreased insulin sensitivity from the fat, so the effect is extra hazardous for metabolic health and predisposes people to metabolic diseases. High amounts of saturated fat and carbs just happen to be found in ice cream, burgers, candy, pastries, and pizza, which are, of course, very popular but

## AN EPIDEMIC OF METABOLIC DISEASE

About a third of the United States has metabolic syndrome, which is a combination of abdominal obesity, high blood pressure, high lipids, and insulin resistance.[10] According to the mitochondrial scientists, metabolic diseases emerge when mitochondrial energy capacity declines past 50 percent, which is the threshold for insufficient energy availability. Without enough energy, the body loses its ability to maintain normal homeostatic end points, i.e., blood sugar, blood pressure, and blood fats within normal ranges. Nearly 50 percent of U.S. adults have high blood pressure,[11] 38 percent have prediabetes,[12] and 12 percent have high cholesterol. These are all signs of metabolism breaking down. Eventually, these risk factors can result in full-blown metabolic diseases (conditions that compromise the normal metabolism of food to energy), such as diabetes, heart disease, dementia, and the most common cancers, like breast, colon, and prostate. As of now, 11 percent of U.S. adults have diabetes,[13] 10.7 percent of those over sixty-five have Alzheimer's,[14] and 25 percent of deaths in the U.S. are due to heart disease.[15] The problems we see on a cellular level are manifesting on a macro level.

problematic foods that make up a large proportion of the Standard American Diet.

Saturated fats have been part of the human diet for two million years, while refined carbs have been in our diets for only about two hundred years, but some people really are more sensitive to saturated fat than others. This is where personalization comes in. While some can eat all the saturated fat they want without any health repercussions, other people can develop dangerously high lipid levels. This can be genetic. I happen to be someone who is genetically sensitive to saturated fat. I know this because I did genetic testing and found I have one copy of a gene variant, called ApoE4, that increases the risk for high cholesterol, heart disease, and Alzheimer's disease. This gene indicates impaired fat metabolism.

THE BEST: Omega-3 fatty acids are the most important fats for your health. These are the fats you get from fatty fish and that your body can synthesize from the fats in chia seeds, flaxseeds, hemp seeds, and walnuts. Omega-3s are especially beneficial for brain health. A 2021 randomized controlled clinical trial[16] in humans demonstrated that approximately 3.4 grams of pharmaceutical-grade EPA/DHA fish oil a day led to significantly better cognitive function, including verbal fluency, language, memory, and visual-motor coordination, over a thirty-month period (the median age of trial participants was sixty-three). I take around 4 grams of Norwegian pharmaceutical-grade fish oil a day because of its neuroprotective benefits.

Research has also shown that regular fish oil consumption lowers the risk of premature death, cardiovascular disease, heart disease, and stroke. It reduces markers of inflammation, improves insulin resistance, and reduces arterial plaque.[17] I think one of the secrets to how I beat my ADHD and achieved better brain function than I ever had before was getting my omegas properly balanced.

Omega-6 fatty acids are necessary too, but because these are the

## NEXT-LEVEL LIPID TESTING

To find out whether you are sensitive to saturated fats, take any genetic test that is widely available online to get your raw data, or get one that specifically looks at health or dietary requirements. You can run your raw data through various programs to analyze your genetic profile in terms of what you should eat. This can give you information about what kinds of fats are best for you from a genetic perspective, as well as how well you do with carbs and how likely you are to have problems metabolizing certain vitamins, like D and $B_{12}$. For more information on getting these tests, go to my website. If you discover that you have one or two copies of the ApoE4 variant, you need to be careful with saturated fats. If you have two copies of the normal ApoE3 variant, or one or two copies of the ApoE2 variant, saturated fats are less problematic for you and you can eat more of them without your LDL ("bad") cholesterol going too high.

If you are concerned about your cholesterol, I recommend getting your NMR lipoprotein profile checked. You may have to order your own online or see a functional doctor or naturopath to get this test. This test goes beyond LDL and HDL cholesterol by looking into particle size, since different particle sizes have different effects. LDL cholesterol, the type generally labeled as "bad cholesterol," is actually made up of two different kinds of particles. Pattern A particles are like bouncy beach balls, and they don't get lodged in your blood vessels as easily. Pattern B particles are like BBs that can get stuck in your arterial wall and contribute to plaques, so B particles are more concerning.

If you want to know your heart disease risk, other important tests are the high-sensitivity C-reactive protein (hs-CRP) and homocysteine. These tests measure markers of inflammation and oxidative stress. If your hs-CRP is greater than 0.5 and your homocysteine is greater than 7, it's time to change your diet and start taking B-vitamins (especially $B_{12}$ and folate) to get these numbers into a healthy range.

fats in many foods people tend to overeat (like most vegetable oils, conventionally raised meat and eggs, and processed foods), we tend to get too much of them. We all need omega-6 and omega-3 fatty acids, but our hunter-gatherer ancestors probably got a balance of about 1:1

or at most 3:1. Now many people have a 30:1 ratio of omega-6 to omega-3,[18] and this balance becomes inflammatory.[19]

Eating more omega-3s can help to rebalance your lipids, induce neurogenesis,[20] and reduce the risk of heart disease,[21] and when women take in more omega-3 fatty acids during pregnancy, it can improve the metabolic health of their child. A 2020 study showed that the benefits outweighed the risks of mercury exposure from fish for pregnant women.[22] Other studies have shown that fish oil can reduce inflammation, improve insulin resistance, reduce plaque in arteries,[23] and improve night vision by 25 percent.[24] I consider this so important for health that I test omega fatty acid balance in all my patients.

## Protein

We eat a lot more protein than we did a hundred years ago, and people who consume large quantities of meat tend to have elevated fasting glucose and increased risk for diabetes,[25] particularly people with higher body mass index, according to studies on meat consumption and risk for elevated blood sugar and diabetes.[26] This surprises many people who think blood sugar is only impacted by carbs. Some proteins are glycolytic, meaning they get metabolized down the carbohydrate pathway, and other proteins are ketogenic, meaning they get metabolized down the protein pathway. Still others can be metabolized through both pathways. Protein gets used first for cellular building blocks, but the excess gets metabolized and can be used as fuel.

I think it's important to be aware of how much protein you are getting and to be careful with your protein source. Organic, grass-fed, pastured sources of animal protein contain more omega-3s and are much less inflammatory than meat from conventional CAFO (confined animal feeding operation) sources, where animals subsist largely on corn- and soybean-based diets, and may also be fed leftover waste

## OPTIMIZING YOUR OMEGAS

A simple blood test can determine your omega 6:3 ratio, balance of EPA and DHA, and levels of other fatty acids, like alpha-linolenic acid (ALA, a plant-based form of omega-3). Ask your doctor about getting your fatty acid levels tested to determine whether your diet is keeping your omegas balanced.

Why does this matter so much? Recent large human prospective and randomized controlled studies show that having sufficient omega-3 fatty acids is associated with lower mortality from all causes and cardiovascular disease, and that they can improve cognitive function and brain structure, increase muscle mass, reduce chronic inflammation, and bolster mitochondrial function in both young and older humans.

A very interesting recent pilot trial also showed that 5 grams daily of pharmaceutical-grade EPA/DHA downregulated aging-related signaling networks in middle-aged women on an epigenetic level.[27] EPA/DHA fatty acids are also precursors to very potent/powerful metabolites that include specialized pro-resolving mediators (often called SPMs) that resolve and counteract age-related chronic inflammation. They may also improve tissue regeneration.

Most randomized controlled trials have used very potent pharmaceutical-grade omega-3 that is highly concentrated, purified, and free of environmental pollutants, and that have very low oxidation levels. Most omega-3 supplements on the market are unfortunately of questionable quality and may not be safe to consume over time and in higher doses. They likely do not have the potent biological effects of pharmaceutical grade omega-3 (with 85 percent omega-3 concentration or above).

And eating large amounts of fatty fish/seafood may lead to long-term adverse health effects. A large prospective study of Swedish women showed that EPA/DHA intake was associated with 80 percent lower risk of skin cancer (melanoma) but that exposure to environmental pollutants (PCBs), mainly from fatty fish, was associated with a four-fold increased risk of malignant melanoma.[28] Speak with your doctor to see if you can be prescribed pharmaceutical omega-3. Real pharmaceutical grade omega-3 may also be available as supplements in certain cases—check my website for updates on which brands I like.

products from food, beverage, and candy factories as a cheap alternative for fattening and finishing.[29]

Another thing we should certainly be avoiding is processed meats like bacon, sausage, deli meats, and cured meats. Large studies in the U.S. and Europe and meta-analyses of epidemiological studies have shown that long-term consumption of processed meat is associated with type-2 diabetes as well as cardiovascular disease and colorectal cancer in both women and men.[30]

To get enough protein, especially if you're trying to limit your saturated fat intake, choose mostly lean sources, like lean cuts of beef, fish, shellfish, leaner poultry, and wild game, like venison and elk. Liver is one of the most nutrient-dense health foods on earth and contains a form of vitamin D that is extremely bioavailable.

Eggs are another high-quality source of protein, especially if they are from pastured chickens (not just "cage free," which often means they are stuck crammed into a barn with an open window). Pastured eggs are more nutrient-rich. Researchers have tested the nutrient content of pastured eggs and found that pastured eggs contain twice the omega-3 fatty acids as conventional eggs[31] and have more concentrated vitamin A. Eggs also contain choline, an essential nutrient that is necessary to make the neurotransmitter acetylcholine, which is vital for brain function, especially if you are at risk of developing Alzheimer's disease.[32] The average egg intake is about 3.8 eggs per week for women and 5.9 eggs per week for men, but some people I know eat many more than this. The research shows that 1 egg per day probably has no adverse effects on cardiometabolic health,[33] but you don't need more than that.

I also believe in being cautious with excess dairy consumption, even if you aren't sensitive to dairy. Dairy can be inflammatory for some people and hard to digest. If you notice you get bloated, have increased mucus production, or have digestive problems after eating dairy, it may be a sign to scale back. I have noticed that when I eat dairy in certain countries, like Israel, I get way fewer symptoms than from dairy in the U.S. I think this is because a lot of the dairy in those countries is made locally and isn't processed to have a long shelf life or be transported across hundreds of miles. Raw-milk cheeses from Europe and those made from goat and sheep's milk are generally the easiest to digest. Raw dairy is available in the United States as well, but you may need to search a bit harder to find it.

There are also plenty of sources of plant proteins. Despite what some say about the dangers of beans and lentils, I'm a fan of them as a source of protein and fiber. That said, many people with autoimmune issues find that beans are a big problem for them. I often recommend patients experiment with a bean-and-grain-free diet if they have autoimmunity. I feel the same about protein powder, which is often pea based. Plant protein powders for me are hit-or-miss. Notice how you feel after you try different protein powders to determine what works for you.

## WHAT ABOUT LECTINS?

Lectins are anti-nutrient proteins that bind to carbohydrates and keep you from absorbing some of the nutrients in food. They are one component of plants that contributes to their xenohormetic effect (page 38), although some people claim they do more harm than good. They are a pathogen that plants use to protect themselves from fungi or from being eaten by insects[34] or animals, so they are poisonous in a way, and in some humans, they might increase risk for autoimmune disease. However, most foods contain some lectins, and for most people, lectins aren't that problematic, especially if you pressure-cook high-lectin foods. Pressure cooking denatures the lectins, so break out your pressure cooker and don't worry or use fear of lectins as an excuse to skip eating your vegetables! But, as I have said before, if you have an autoimmune condition, experiment with going lectin-free and see how you feel.

## Micronutrients and Phytonutrients

Micronutrients are vitamins and minerals, and they are critically important because micronutrient density is one of the keys to longevity and energy production. We used to get plenty of micronutrients from fruits and vegetables, but our soil quality is declining significantly, depleted due to industrial agriculture.[35] Now we're importing more than half of our produce, and imported produce is much less micronutrient-dense than fresh local produce because shipping and storing reduces micronutrient content. In order to get enough micronutrients to fuel your mitochondria, you should make grass-fed, pasture-raised animal products and fresh produce the foundation of your diet. I also like shellfish, nuts, and seeds for their nutrient density. If you can, try to get as much produce as possible from local or organic producers, and source your meat and fish from quality suppliers. I aim for grass-fed and wild sources of protein as much as I can. There may be a lot of controversy around carnivore and vegan diets, but having looked into the literature on this, I have concluded that omnivorous diets create the highest likelihood for longevity and reproductive success.[36]

Phytonutrients are substances in plants that aren't vitamins or minerals but that have been identified as beneficial to health. You can identify produce rich in phytonutrients by color:

- **RED, ORANGE, AND YELLOW** vegetables and fruits have a lot of carotenoids. I've found in my research and personal experience that eating more carotenoids can have an actual, noticeable effect on skin quality and appearance. One study showed that carotenoid-rich diets resulted in a more pleasing appearance and better-smelling sweat.[37]

- **GREEN** vegetables provide all sorts of cancer cell inhibitors like zeaxanthin, isothiocyanates, and lutein. I'm also a big fan of high quality spirulina and chlorella tablets that contain superoxide dismutase (SOD) and chlorophyll, which are profound antioxidants that directly protect the mitochondria from free radicals.

- **BLUE AND PURPLE** vegetables often have anthocyanins in them, which may delay aging and help with heart functioning and the prevention of blood clots.

- **WHITE AND BROWN** vegetables like onions, garlic, and mushrooms contain allicin, which has anti-tumor properties. White fruits and vegetables often also contain quercetin and kaempferol. Quercetin is particularly helpful as an antiviral.

## Personalizing Nutrition

A lot of people ask me: Should I be an omnivore? Carnivore? Herbivore? Vegan? Paleo? Keto? My response is this: I don't like to label or limit nutrition, and I believe we should focus less on trends and more on getting nutrient density and diversity from a variety of animals and plants. So yes, in some ways you could say that I am pro-omnivore. I think one reason why so many nutritionists and experts disagree about the best way to eat is because different people do well on different diets. The field of nutrition is ever evolving, and there is always controversy around metabolic health and proper macronutrient ratios and food sourcing.

When I started looking at diets to treat metabolic diseases like diabetes, I noticed that multiple approaches were working. Both high-fat ketogenic diets, which lower carbohydrate intake and insulin output, and low-fat vegan diets, which lower fat intake to improve insulin resistance by lowering HbA1c (a marker of blood sugar over time), led to weight loss. Both were effective at improving metabolic health because they both focused on whole foods, removed processed foods, and limited overeating. If you limit the biggest culprits of metabolic disease from the diet (e.g., ultra-processed foods, fast foods, refined carbs, fried vegetable oils, processed meat, and sugar), you're going to see improvements.

We know humans can adapt to variable whole-food supplies. What matters is maintaining consistency with dietary changes. Sometimes following a restricted diet can make compliance easier, but that's not for everyone, either.

In terms of biomarkers, if you look at the high-carb, low-fat vegan people, they tend to have higher triglycerides but lower cholesterol overall, including lower LDL and lower HDL. The effect on glucose varies, but in general, higher-carb diets do seem to increase insulin output. But that can depend on diet quality. With a lower fat intake, this dietary pattern still improves insulin sensitivity, resulting in a lower blood sugar level overall. People who eat high-carb vegan diets also tend to have a much better blood sugar response to carbohydrates because they are more carb-adapted, but they have a harder time switching into fat burning. They aren't always metabolically flexible.

For low-carb people, which would include the Paleo-keto-ancestral group, they tend to have lower triglycerides and higher HDL cholesterol, but some people get high LDL cholesterol. People on these diets tend to have lower glucose levels, and they get lower post-meal blood sugar and lower fasting glucose. The problem is that the moment people who are eating ketogenic eat any carbohydrates, their blood sugar spikes. They can lose their carbohydrate adaptation, also becoming metabolically inflexible.

Different diets simply work differently for every individual, partly due to genetics and partly due to each person's microbiome composition. This isn't a new idea. You may remember back when everyone talked about mesomorphs, ectomorphs, and endomorphs. These were three body types that supposedly did best on different kinds of diets.

This idea is even present in the ancient Indian health system, Ayurveda, that types people as being predominantly vata, pitta, or kapha, which are both body types and temperaments.

The way I see it, people who are highly active, or naturally slender, or naturally have a fast metabolism, tend to do better with the higher-carb diets. People who are more sedentary or who have a larger build seem to do better on more ancestral diets with fewer carbs, and they seem to enjoy these diets more. People who are in the middle—naturally somewhere in between lean and muscular—do best on a whole foods balanced diet with a mix of carbohydrates and fats.

Put simply, I think it's probably true that different people adapt best to different diets. This may explain why some people rave about their vegan diet fixing their health problems while others rave about their keto or paleo diet helping them thrive. When you find a diet that works for your type, it feels great and you can't imagine it wouldn't work for everyone. I've tried all these diets at some point in my life, and I've settled somewhere between—low-carb and balanced. I periodically wear a continuous glucose monitor (page 129) and track my body's response to sugar and carbohydrates. Tracking blood sugar and noticing how you feel in response to different foods can help you figure out what works for your body. I discovered that my body does best with a lower carb intake, but I don't thrive on being continuously in ketosis.

I've become so attuned to my body that I am no longer in a battle with it (as I was when I was younger and felt I needed to starve myself to be a size 2). It's super important to point out that if you implement different tracking technologies and find yourself obsessing over food or developing orthorexia (page 49) or an eating disorder, then it's time to take a step back and examine your relationship to yourself.

After I spent a year focusing on self-love and healing attachment wounds, my relationship to food changed because I healed my relationship to myself and my parents. I know how different foods affect me and I no longer beat myself up for indulging. When my body is under stress, it holds onto calories, which I now understand is a protective response and a way for my body to store fuel in anticipation of future challenges. When it's relaxed, the pounds come off because my body knows it's safe. I've learned to love my body whether it is curvy or lean and learned to listen to what it needs to feel healthy.

## Dietary Dogma

When you find a diet that works for your type, it feels great and you can't imagine it wouldn't work for everyone, at all life stages. But the funny thing about bodies is that they are both unique and changing all the time. There are many anecdotal stories of people who had major improvements on ketogenic or vegan diets, but after they lost weight or developed nutritional deficiencies, they shifted to a more balanced diet and achieved even better health. Don't be afraid to experiment and change your diet when something is no longer working. Dietary dogma isn't conducive to the dynamic nature of health.

If you subscribe to a diet that eliminates major food groups, whether that's animal products or all grains and beans, it's important to get your labs checked occasionally. You may find deficiencies or imbalances. I know a lot of people who were 100 percent plant based and eventually switched back to eating animal products after developing several micronutrient deficiencies, especially omega-3s and vitamin $B_{12}$. It is possible to avoid micronutrient deficiencies if you keep track and adjust your food and supplements as needed, but it's certainly easier to get everything you need if you are more omnivorous.

On the other side, someone doing keto may do great initially and lose excess weight, but they often become metabolically inflexible and unable to tolerate carbohydrates without huge blood sugar spikes. Eventually, they switch back to eating some carbs and feel better than they did doing keto long-term.

An extreme vegan, carnivore, or ketogenic diet can be good therapeutically in the short term because rules can help people stay consistent. But, they may not be so good in the long term. If you need to go vegan or keto temporarily to get your body on track, great, but stay flexible. If you need to change what you do because your body is no longer reacting well to that diet, it's okay not to stick with the same pattern forever.

Some signals that your diet isn't working (or is no longer working) include hair loss, nail problems, mood problems, focus problems, and other issues with brain function. These are all signs that your nutrition is inadequate. Often the culprit is that people aren't eating enough vegetables—and that translates to insufficient micronutrients and phytonutrients. Even vegans, who may rely heavily on refined carbs, processed foods, and soy, can have this problem.

Some people say they have a hard time digesting vegetables, but this is a bit of a catch-22: that intolerance is often a result of low vegetable intake. When you don't get enough plant-based fiber, your microbiome suffers, and so does your ability to digest vegetables and absorb micronutrients and phytonutrients. We'll talk more about the microbiome in chapter 8, but for now it's just important to understand that the more you avoid eating vegetables, the less able you will be able to tolerate them.

Biohacking is about self-experimentation, so try on different dietary styles and pay attention to how your body responds. Do you have more energy or less? Do you feel more pain or less? Do you feel happier or less happy? Food can have a noticeable effect on physical and mental health, but you have to pay attention to notice it. If you do this, over time, you'll learn what works for you.

And if you need support, look for personalized nutrition counseling from a functional medicine doctor who can run labs for food sensitivities in particular. I recommend an elimination diet (see "How to Do an Elimination Diet," page 269, for how to do this) at least once for every patient, regardless of their health status. It's the gold-standard diagnostic test for identifying the most common food intolerances, like eggs, soy, dairy, wheat, nuts, beans, and legumes, and it's just one more tool for helping you determine the right diet for your body, your genetics, your needs, and your lifestyle.

## DIETARY BIOHACKS IN THIS CHAPTER

- Use a food tracker to keep track of your fiber, sugar, macronutrient, and micronutrient intake.

- Get a genetic test to determine your ApoE status, to check whether you are sensitive to saturated fats.

- Ask your doctor about getting an NMR profile for advanced cholesterol testing, to get more information about your cholesterol levels.

- Avoid refined grains and lean into more whole grains, or reduce grain intake altogether if you notice it makes you feel better.

- Experiment going on and off of lectins to see how you feel.

- Test your hs-CRP and homocysteine to check for inflammation and oxidative stress. If these are high, add B-vitamins to your supplement regimen.

- Test your omega fatty acid balance. If your omega-3 fatty acids are too low, eat more fatty fish and consider supplementing with medical-grade fish oil.

- Cut back on vegetable oil! Replace it with fruit oils like olive and avocado oils.

- Quit processed meat and default to lean animal and plant protein sources.

- Supplement with choline if you don't eat eggs.

- Don't eat more than an egg a day if you do eat eggs.

- Test micronutrient and phytonutrient status to see if you have deficiencies.

- Test your genes to determine any genetic influences on your ideal diet.

- Consider food sensitivity testing.

- Experiment with different dietary patterns to find out what works best and feels best for you.

# CHAPTER 7

# Blood Sugar Is the Ultimate Energy Biomarker

In 2012 about 56 million people died throughout the world; 620,000 of them died due to human violence (war killed 120,000 people, and crime killed another 500,000). In contrast, 800,000 committed suicide, and 1.5 million died of diabetes. Sugar is now more dangerous than gunpowder.

—Yuval Noah Harari

The fluctuations of your blood sugar and insulin on a day-to-day and hour-to-hour basis are, in my opinion, the ultimate biomarkers. Blood sugar influences how you use energy or store it as fat, how well you repair and heal, how much inflammation you have, and to a large extent, whether or not you will eventually develop a chronic disease.

Briefly, here's how it works: in response to the digestion of food and the release of glucose into the bloodstream, the pancreas releases the hormone insulin, and like a key, insulin unlocks the glucose receptors in cells, opening the door to let the glucose inside the cells, where the mitochondria can use it to make energy in the form of ATP. If you eat a little bit of food and your blood sugar goes up a small amount, you'll get a dose of insulin, which enables the glucose to be taken into the cells. If you eat too much, or you eat a meal high in refined carbs and sugar, the surge of glucose in your bloodstream will require a commensurate amount of insulin to enable the glucose to be utilized by the cells. Eat a lot of carbs, and your body releases a lot of insulin.

Insulin sends glucose into the cells, including into muscle and liver cells, for short-term storage as glycogen, and into fat cells for long-term storage. But with consistent overeating, or as I call it, overfueling, cells flooded with extra glucose start to become resistant to insulin's cell-unlocking features. The cells stay locked, so glucose can't get in. This prompts the pancreas to release even more insulin, to try to get the cells to open. This may work for a while, but eventually, cells become more and more stubbornly locked. They are trying to stem the tide of incoming fuel because it's too much. Essentially, the cell is saying, "I can't take up the amount of fuel you're trying to force inside me! Stop pouring in fuel! I can't make the energy to metabolize it. I need a break!" This is insulin resistance.

Consistently overeating causes a buildup of fat cells because the

## INSULIN RESISTANCE AS AN ADAPTATION

Why would our bodies stop recognizing insulin? Scientists posit that it's an adaptive response. If an early human was exposed to a famine, their body would quickly adapt to the low food supply by switching to burning fat and making cells less sensitive to insulin, so that any sugar that was available could get to the brain rather than getting locked up in fat cells.

But that doesn't work well in a modern environment that is high stress with constant availability of high-carb food. High stress used to coincide with low food availability, but now we have high stress coinciding with high food availability. You can be eating a lot, with plenty of glucose coming in, but because you're stressed, your body anticipates you might starve later, so it stores as much fat as it can and leaves sugar in your blood in case your brain needs it. Then and now, stress hormones increase insulin resistance.

fuel you're not immediately using must go somewhere. The first storage spots for excess fat and glucose are the liver and skeletal muscle cells. Glucose is first stored in the form of glycogen for easy access. Once those storage locations are full, the next storage spot is your fat cells, in subcutaneous tissue (tissue beneath your skin). The body takes extra glucose and combines it with fatty acids to form a triglyceride molecule, which gets stored in fat cells.

Once all the subcutaneous adipose tissue gets filled up with fuel, extra fat spills into the viscera and starts to crowd the organs. *Ectopic* means "abnormal place or position," so ectopic fat is fat that gets stored in and around the liver, skeletal muscle, vasculature, heart, or pancreas, where it is definitely not meant to be. One of the biggest predictors of dangerous visceral fat storage is simply overeating (overfueling), and you don't have to be overweight or obese for this to happen. Plenty of skinny people overeat and spill fat (fuel) into their viscera, causing metabolic disease. This is known as TOFI: thin outside, fat inside.

When a cell is overfilled with fuel, the mitochondria are also impacted. They can become overwhelmed with too much fuel and can malfunction and stop working. Essentially, overfueling "breaks" the mitochondria, and in turn, broken mitochondria can make the cell less insulin sensitive in a variety of ways. First, dysfunctional mitochondria have reduced energy output (less ATP for the body to use to process glucose and make insulin). Second, the backup of excess fuel and reduced ability to process that fuel create an increase in reactive oxygen species—that inflammatory byproduct of fuel production that's like the exhaust from a car in a garage. This combination of less energy and more inflammation-causing "exhaust" can interfere with insulin's ability to do its job. The whole system starts to break down because there's just too much fuel and exhaust everywhere. It's not how the body is supposed to function.

As blood sugar continues to rise, your mitochondrial power plants are further damaged, and the cycle continues. This dysfunction will start to manifest as prediabetes, which occurs when blood sugar gets slightly higher than normal. The higher the blood sugar goes, the more the cells in the pancreas (called beta cells) that produce insulin get worn out and stop working. By the time you're prediabetic, you've lost about 40 percent of your beta cell function. By the time you're diabetic, you've lost over 60 percent of your beta cell function.[1]

This is why blood sugar gets so high when someone becomes diabetic. They've lost the ability to produce enough insulin to keep blood sugar in the normal range. As blood sugar wreaks havoc all over your body, it can cause serious damage to both the small and large blood vessels and nerves. The more blood sugar spikes you experience, the more

## OPTIMIZE BLOOD SUGAR AND INSULIN FOR BETTER SKIN

Chronic high blood sugar isn't only damaging to your pancreas; it's also damaging to your skin. High blood sugar accelerates skin aging through a process called glycation. Sugar attaches to proteins, fats, and DNA in the body, and everything gets "sticky." It attaches to collagen and breaks it down, reducing your skin's elasticity and resilience, resulting in wrinkling and aging. Imagine browning sugar in a pan until it burns—glycation is a little like that browning reaction. It's like cooking your skin. Simply eating a diet low in sugar and refined carbs can prevent this process and keep your skin looking younger for longer.

A lesser-known effect of too much insulin is the stimulation of oil-producing glands in the skin, contributing to acne. A lot of women still get adult acne but addressing blood sugar and insulin problems can help to resolve it. People often think that acne can only be addressed through topical treatments, but it's far more effective to address through diet and lifestyle.

Throughout my teens and twenties, I had a lot of problems with back acne. I worked really hard on my blood sugar metabolism, and I also drastically cut back on dairy products because dairy has insulin-stimulating properties. These two interventions completely resolved my acne. The beautiful thing about our skin is that it's a window into our bodies. If we see our skin change, it means something inside us has changed.

exhaust fumes (reactive oxygen species) come off your cells and damage the lining of your blood vessels, making them stiff and contributing to the development of hypertension. Because of blood vessel damage, people with diabetes often suffer from vision loss, heart disease, and reduced blood flow to extremities, which can lead to amputation. What's more, both insulin resistance and mitochondrial dysfunction are implicated in chronic disease states like obesity, type 2 diabetes, high blood pressure, high cholesterol, and cardiovascular disease, as well as some forms of cancer and dementia. This is how high blood sugar destroys the body.

The origin of metabolic dysfunction is clear: when you break the engines of the cells, metabolism breaks down and diseases emerge.

## Using a Continuous Glucose Monitor

One of the best biohacking inventions of the century in my opinion is a device that can help you understand what your blood sugar is doing in real time, all the time. It's the continuous glucose monitor (CGM). This device doesn't require sticking your finger to measure your blood sugar, like people with diabetes have had to do for decades. Instead, you wear a disk on your upper arm that measures the blood sugar in your interstitial fluid all the time, so you can find out, via an app on your phone, what your blood sugar is doing—first thing in the morning, before and after meals, last thing at night, or whenever you want to check it. This is a great way to understand in real time how foods and other activities like exercise, hydration, stress, and sleep affect your blood sugar, since different foods and lifestyles have different effects on different people.

CGMs are still new and still mostly only available by prescription. Your doctor might prescribe one for you if you are prediabetic (as so many people are), but even if you aren't, you might be able to get one if you have a family history of blood sugar problems or are overweight. Right now, there are companies working on making CGMs available without a prescription, for biohackers, athletes, or anyone who wants one, and I don't think it will be much longer before you can buy one over the counter.

There are various models and each comes with its own instructions—check out my website for more information on the different options and how best to use them. No matter which option you choose, I recommend that you keep a food diary and track the impact of foods and combinations of foods on your blood sugar. Note how you feel after eating, so you can understand your symptoms in terms of your blood sugar data. When you ate that granola bar or that watermelon, was your energy low or high? Are you craving more sweets? Are you thirsty or hungry? Are you having problems concentrating or are you in the zone? Are you irritable? Cheerful? Are you having any physical symptoms, like bloating, reflux, or a headache?

If you notice a favorite food spikes your blood sugar, try eating a smaller portion, having a tablespoon of apple cider vinegar in water before your meal, or eating it at the end of your meal to slow down the spike. If some of these strategies work, you'll know how to eat that food. If none of them work, you'll get the message that this food probably isn't a fit for you, even if it's a food generally considered to be healthy.

The CGM is a tool to help you bring more attention to your body's reactions and feedback, so you can personalize your diet to match your body's needs and reactions. You won't need to wear it forever. After wearing a CGM off and on over a few years, I am now able to tell when my blood sugar is high, low, or normal, just by how I feel. I thought I was healthy in 2014 when I first started tracking my blood glucose, but I discovered that I was on my way to developing prediabetes. My blood sugar was hitting above 140 regularly after meals, and it was right below 100 fasting, so I knew I needed to do something to turn things around.

I've learned that when my fasting blood sugar hovers around 80 to 85 and when my postprandial (post-meal) blood sugar is consistently below 120 mg/dL, I don't get tired during the day, I don't have as many cravings, my skin doesn't break out, I don't have mood swings, I have easier periods, and I just feel better. If I wait until my blood sugar is below 85 before meals, then I know I'm definitely going to be hungry enough to eat. If I do get a spike in my blood sugar from eating high-carb foods, I know I'll be on the glycemic roller coaster for hours, which will make me feel hungry, tired, and irritable. Using a CGM with intention and keen observation can teach you more about what your body is doing than just about any other biohacking device.

## How to Interpret Your Blood Sugar Numbers

According to the CDC,[2] normal fasting blood sugar (when you first wake up in the morning before eating) is 99 mg/dL or lower. If your fasting blood sugar is 100 to 125 mg/dL, that's considered prediabetes.[3] If it's 126 mg/dL or higher, that indicates diabetes.

But a lot of biohackers, as well as integrative medicine practitioners, think those numbers are too high. I'd personally rather see your fasting blood sugar around 85 mg/dL (plus or minus 7 mg/dL). That said, there is a limit to how low you should go. If you regularly reach a level below 70 mg/dL, that's stressful on your body, too. This is mostly a concern for elderly populations, who can become easily undernourished.

Tracking your blood sugar response after eating can help you determine which foods and how much food puts you into the danger zone. The general rule is that glucose shouldn't rise above 140 mg/dL during the two hours after eating. Most people experience blood sugar levels of 99 to 137 after a meal, but some people think this is even too high. The American Academy of Clinical Endocrinologists recommends that post-meal blood sugar be less than 120 after two hours. Some research suggests cardiovascular risks increase at 160 mg/dL after eating due to the fact that blood sugar this high damages small blood vessels. Your kidneys are also filled with tiny blood vessels that can become damaged by high blood sugar. You may start spilling sugar into your urine when your blood sugar after meals goes above 160. This blood vessel damage can also lead to heart disease, cancer, strokes, and dementia.

## INSULIN TESTING

A fasting insulin test is harder to get than a blood sugar test. It's not a test doctors normally do, but I always recommend it because a high fasting insulin level, even in the presence of a normal fasting blood sugar reading, can be a warning sign that you are developing insulin resistance. Insulin sensitivity can begin to decline ten to thirteen years before blood sugar is dysregulated enough for a diagnosis.

Fasting insulin has also been identified as a test that can more accurately predict prediabetes. Normal fasting insulin according to most standard lab ranges is considered <25 mIU/mL. Yet, a study of 965 women with obesity, 29.7 percent of whom had prediabetes, showed that fasting insulin levels above 9 mIU/mL correctly identified prediabetes in most of the affected patients.[4] The average insulin level in the U.S. is 8.4 mIU/mL for women and 8.8 for men, which means a lot of people are right on the cusp of prediabetes and don't even know it.[5]

I have patients with normal post-meal glucose on a CGM, but their insulin levels were 11 mIU/mL and they had symptoms of insulin resistance (e.g., energy problems, acne, sugar cravings, feeling tired after high-carb meals, and low-level depression). Too much insulin in your blood is a sign that you may be eating too many carbs for your body to handle. I'd much rather see a level below 6 mIU/mL.

Here are some benchmarks to help you interpret and keep track of your data:

*Fasting glucose*
- DIABETES DIAGNOSIS: ≥ 126 mg/dL
- PREDIABETES: ≥ 100mg/dL
- GOOD: < 100 mg/dL
- BETTER: < 90 mg/dL
- BEST: < 85 mg/dL

*Peak post-meal glucose (the peak typically happens between 46 and 60 minutes after eating)*
- SUGAR SPILLING INTO URINE: 160–180 mg/dL
- DAMAGE TO SMALL BLOOD VESSELS: > 160 mg/dL
- DAMAGE TO LARGE BLOOD VESSELS: > 135 mg/dL
- HEALTHY: < 120 mg/dL

*Two hours after eating*
- TYPE 2 DIABETES: > 200 mg/dL
- PREDIABETES: > 140 mg/dL
- GOOD: 140 mg/dL
- BETTER: < 125 mg/dL
- BEST: < 110 mg/dL

*Average daily glucose (mean 24-hour glucose)*
- 79–100 MG/DL (BEST)
- 89–104 MG/DL (NORMAL)

*Recommended range for your blood sugar tracking app settings*
- 72–110 MG/DL (IDEAL)
- 70–140 MG/DL (NORMAL)

*Fasting Insulin*
- STANDARD REFERENCE RANGE: <25 mIU/mL
- GOOD: < 9 mIU/mL
- BETTER: < 8 mIU/mL
- BEST: < 6 mIU/mL

## How to Bring Down Your CGM Numbers

If after wearing a CGM you find that your blood sugar is going too high after meals, there are some easy ways to get your numbers into a healthy range. Let's start with some basic food hacks for avoiding big blood sugar spikes:

- **AVOID REFINED CARBOHYDRATES AND SUGAR.** The biggest culprits here are white carbs (found in flour-based foods like pastries, muffins, pizza, and bread), processed potatoes (like fries and chips), and sugar (e.g., in desserts, candy, and many processed foods and condiments).

- **EAT LOW-GLYCEMIC-INDEX FOODS.** The glycemic index is a measure of how high a food spikes an average person's blood sugar (it's the average of one thousand people's glycemic response to a single food), with 0 being something that doesn't spike at all, such as water, and 100 being the effect of pure glucose. Anything over 70 is considered high-glycemic. The average person can lower their blood sugar meaningfully just by lowering their intake of high-glycemic foods. It isn't always easy to guess what constitutes a high-glycemic food, but there are plenty of free lists available online.

- **EAT FRESH FRUIT INSTEAD OF DRIED.** Dried fruit can have a blood sugar effect as extreme as candy. Opt for fresh fruit instead.

- **DRINK VINEGAR WATER BEFORE EATING.** Adding a tablespoon of vinegar to a glass of water and drinking it before you eat a meal is a simple way to lower your blood sugar, especially if you know you'll be eating a carbohydrate-rich meal. Vinegar can activate AMPK (AMP-activated kinase), a protein that acts like a fuel gauge for cells and has been shown, when activated, to have a positive effect on blood sugar, in a way similar to the diabetes medication metformin or the herb berberine.[6] It could also help with weight loss—according to a small 2014 study, people who took apple cider vinegar before meals while on a low-calorie diet lost more weight after twelve weeks than those on the same diet without the apple cider vinegar.[7]

- **EAT NON-STARCHY VEGETABLES FIRST, PROTEIN SECOND, AND STARCHY CARBS LAST.** One of the best things you can do to mitigate a blood sugar spike is to eat non-starchy vegetables before starchy foods. Eating starchy foods last, when your body is already digesting foods higher in fiber and protein, will slow the rise of blood sugar. In a 2014 review,[8] researchers studied this effect on people with type 2 diabetes and found that postprandial glucose and insulin levels decreased significantly in those patients who ate vegetables before their carbohydrates, compared to patients eating their carbohydrates first. Over the course of the two-and-a-half-year study, patients eating vegetables first had significantly improved glycemic control. Another small study[9] of people who did not have diabetes showed that after fasting overnight, consuming carbohydrates after vegetables and/or meat resulted in lower rises in glucose and insulin after meals than in those who ate the carbohydrates first.

- **DON'T EAT REFINED OR STARCHY CARBOHYDRATES ALONE.** This is a recipe for a blood sugar spike. Pair these foods with protein (e.g., chicken with rice or an apple with peanut butter) to avoid a big spike.

- **MAKE RESISTANT STARCHES.** Cooking can make a starchy food higher glycemic because the more you expose the surface area of a carbohydrate to enzymes, the faster it will be processed into your bloodstream. But if you cook and then cool a starchy vegetable like rice or a potato, some of that starch turns into resistant starch and will have less of a blood sugar effect. That said, I still wouldn't recommend large servings of these foods.

- **SUPPLEMENT FOR BLOOD SUGAR CONTROL.** Berberine, chromium, alpha lipoic acid, vitamin D, resveratrol, gymnema, bitter melon, magnesium, and cinnamon can help stabilize blood sugar. Berberine is the most potent of these; research shows that taking 500 mg two or three times a day (before large meals) has effects on blood sugar similar to the diabetes medication metformin.[10] In another study, forty-eight participants with type 2 diabetes who took berberine for three months had lowered fasting and postprandial blood sugar starting after just one week, which lasted to the end of the trial. They also had lowered HbA1c, lowered fasting insulin, and significant drops in total and LDL cholesterol. The researchers concluded that berberine was a potent hypoglycemic agent with beneficial effects on fat metabolism.

- **EXERCISE BEFORE AND/OR AFTER EATING.** This is one of the most effective tips for dealing with postprandial blood sugar. Exercise increases oxidative capacity and the uptake of glucose into the muscle without insulin's help, so you can fuel without insulin output. The more you exercise, the less insulin you need to lower your blood sugar. A few years ago, I broke a fast with high-fat, high-carb pancakes for breakfast and got a huge, unexpected glucose spike of 187! High-fat, high-carb meals are like metabolic kryptonite. So, I went outside to do yoga in the sun and in thirty-six minutes, I dropped my sugar by 79 points, down to 108.

- **UNDERSTAND EXERCISE-INDUCED BLOOD SUGAR SPIKES.** As long as you haven't consumed some form of sugar-based beverage that could have caused a spike, if you do a hard workout and see a blood sugar spike, it's not a cause for too much concern. Your body is liberating blood sugar to feed your muscles, but the long-term effect is generally beneficial. Still, you may want to watch how often this happens. For example, as I noted earlier, doing too much HIIT (more than 150 minutes per week) can stress the body and tax the mitochondria.

- **WAIT UNTIL YOUR BLOOD SUGAR GOES BELOW 85 MG/DL TO EAT AGAIN.** This is one of my favorite blood sugar hacks. Once you start tracking your blood sugar, you'll know when your body is ready to eat again. This is really helpful if you've lost touch with your body's own hunger and satiety signals, if you tend to eat based on habit or emotions. A study in *Nutrition & Metabolism*[11] showed that waiting until blood sugar goes below 85 mg/dL can train people to recognize true versus conditional hunger.

- **BE CAUTIOUS ABOUT SUGAR-FREE AND GLUTEN-FREE FOODS.** These look healthy on the label but they may be filled with ingredients that spike your blood sugar. For example, maltitol, which is found in a lot of energy bars and sugar-free candy, will spike your blood sugar. Gluten-free ingredients like rice flour are bound to spike your blood sugar because they are rapidly digested into glucose.

These are the most effective lifestyle hacks to bring down whole-body insulin sensitivity, blunt glycemic variability, and lower fasting blood sugar:

- Avoid overeating, and if you are overweight, aim to lose 5 to 7 percent of your body weight.

- Eat a diet rich in high-fiber plants (aim for 25 grams of fiber per day) and polyphenols. To get more polyphenols, eat more colorful vegetables, berries, and fruits, particularly dark berries such as blueberries and blackcurrants; use herbs and spices in cooking, especially turmeric, ginger, cinnamon, garlic, ginseng, rosemary, and fenugreek; drink green tea; and eat raw cacao.

- Avoid sedentary behavior. Move and exercise regularly.

- Avoid the metabolic toxins in processed meat, trans fats, and fried food.

- Avoid the toxins in pollution, alcohol (less than one drink a day), and cigarette smoke.

*To reduce glycemic variability*

- Eat at regular mealtimes and cut back on excessive snacking.

- Work on managing stress, which can cause high glycemic variability.

- If you are stressed or burned out, eat a protein-rich breakfast every day and have a small snack before bed to keep blood sugar steady through the night.

*To reduce fasting glucose*

- Try intermittent fasting (see chapter 9) and stop eating before six P.M. to extend your overnight fast.

- Avoid processed snack food, fast food, and high-fructose corn syrup.

- Increase soluble fiber (e.g., prunes, carrots, and psyllium or acacia fiber) to feed gut bacteria.

- Alternate periods of lower carb and higher carb eating (carb cycling) to increase metabolic flexibility.

- Get sufficient and quality sleep and avoid sleep deprivation.

---

### BLOOD SUGAR BIOHACKS IN THIS CHAPTER

- Reduce overeating and use the fuel you're already carrying around.

- Start tracking your fasting and after-meal blood sugar with a continuous glucose monitor or a standard blood sugar test kit.

- Hack acne and reverse skin aging by reducing refined carbs and sugar in your diet to drop your insulin level below 6 mIU/mL.

- Experiment with a CGM to see what foods spike your blood sugar.

- Use your CGM to see what happens when you intermittently fast, eat different types and amounts of carbohydrates, exercise, and meditate.

- Use what you learn from your CGM to develop a personalized diet and lifestyle.

- Work on getting your fasting glucose, peak post-meal glucose, two-hour post-meal glucose, and average daily glucose into the ideal range.

- Improve your blood sugar levels by eating more low-glycemic foods, choosing fresh fruit over dried fruit, taking a tablespoon of vinegar in water before meals, eating non-starchy vegetables before starchy carbs, and eating refined or starchy carbs with protein, never alone.

- Cook and reheat starchy carbs for more resistant starch to reduce blood sugar spikes.

- Take blood-sugar-lowering supplements, especially 500 mg of berberine two or three times per day. You could also try resveratrol, gymnema, or cinnamon.

- Exercise before and/or after eating to reduce blood sugar spikes.

- Wait until you are hungry to eat, which is usually when your blood sugar drops below 85 mg/dL on your CGM.

# CHAPTER 8

# The Gut-Energy Connection

All disease begins in the gut.

—Hippocrates

Your microbiome is the community of microbes living inside you, most densely in your large intestine. These microbes are mostly bacteria but also include fungi, viruses, and other microbes. Your microbiome assists you with digestion, immunity, blood sugar balance, hormone production, metabolism, metabolic flexibility, and much more. In fact, your microbiome has a hand in most of the major processes of your body. Those microbes live in symbiosis with you—they keep you healthy and you provide them with a place to live.

Pathogenic microbes are in there, too, and they have a place, but they can cause health problems if they overgrow. They can cause digestive issues, inflammation, and problems with metabolism, blood sugar balance, hormones, skin, mood, and more. The good news is that when you eat food rich in nutrients, polyphenols, and fiber, you fuel the growth of the beneficial microbes, and they keep the bad guys in check. However, when you eat junk food high in sugar, vegetable oil, and refined carbs, you fuel the growth of those pathogenic microbes that increase inflammation. So the question is: Which microbes do you want to feed?

Your microbiome influences your metabolism in several important ways. One of those is blood sugar metabolism.[1] Research shows that variations in blood sugar spikes are tied to variations in microbiomes.[2]

Gut microbes influence insulin secretion, short-chain fatty acid production, bile acid metabolism, and fat tissue regulation, all of which can impact glycemic control. Those microbes also affect your appetite, absorption of energy from food, storage of liver fat, gut motility, and lipid metabolism.[3]

The gut microbiome also regulates factors that can affect mitochondrial metabolism and the production of new mitochondria as well as the disposal of dysfunctional mitochondria.[4] For example, when we eat pomegranates, berries, and nuts containing the polyphenols ellagitannins and ellagic acid, our microbiomes convert these into Urolithin A. This molecule improves mitochondrial function, reduces inflammation, and increases mitophagy (throwing out the dysfunctional batteries that have lost their charge), all of which enhance cellular health. Cross-talk between the microbiome and the mitochondria can also contribute to blood sugar dysregulation and diabetes.[5] If your microbiome isn't functioning properly, it's safe to assume that your mitochondria are also suffering some consequences.

When you eat junk foods, part of the inflammatory effect is due to feeding the microbes that increase inflammation in your gut. A poor diet high in sugar and saturated fat and low in fiber and nutrients changes the composition of your microbiome, so the pathogenic microbes have an advantage over the beneficial microbes that should be dominant.[6] A damaged microbiome can impair immunity. The microbiome plays a significant role in training your immune system to react properly to pathogens. We need a healthy microbiome to know what to attack and what to preserve—it knows the difference between a foreign substance, like a virus, and cells that belong to the body. Without this, we risk developing autoimmune conditions, which is what happens when the body attacks itself.

Worsening the issue is a compromised gut barrier caused by inflammation in the digestive tract. This is leaky gut, a.k.a. intestinal permeability. Many things can compromise the gut barrier, causing it to become more permeable: the modern lifestyle influences we've already discussed, antibiotic use, toxins in our environment, other medications (especially antibiotics and NSAIDs like ibuprofen and naproxen), parasitic infections, fungal overgrowth such as candida, ingesting allergenic foods, low stomach acid, and pancreatic insufficiency (not producing enough digestive enzymes), just to name a few. When the gut barrier becomes compromised, food particles and bacterial toxins can leak into the bloodstream. This creates systemic inflammation, which can be a major energy drain and exposes immune cells to food particles, causing the body to start reacting to food as though it's foreign. This is when autoimmune and inflammatory disorders can emerge.[7]

If you struggle with digestive problems like gas, bloating, loose stools, or irritable bowel syndrome, you may have a leaky gut. Other signs of leaky gut syndrome include food intolerances, seasonal allergies,

## HOW LEAKY GUT CAN LEAD TO AUTOIMMUNITY

Genetics combined with environmental insults like stress and infections in the presence of a weakened immune system can trigger the development of autoimmune conditions.[8] Autoimmunity is, essentially, the body's immune system mistakenly attacking itself.

Here's how this works: the body is supposed to maintain what's known as tolerance, meaning it knows the difference between the self and foreign pathogens. Our immune system recognizes certain peptides found on microorganisms that can cause infection, like viruses and bacteria. When our immune cells identify these peptides, they attack them. However, an overactive immune system can get confused when it encounters similar-looking antigens found on the body's own cells, or in undigested food particles that have leaked out of the digestive tract. The body then starts to attack itself—it might target the digestive tract itself, or it may attack and damage nerve cells, skin cells, pancreatic cells, or joint tissue.

eczema, autoimmunity, chronic fatigue syndrome (or just being tired all the time), mood issues like anxiety and depression, problems losing weight despite an excellent diet, achy or swollen joints, trouble concentrating, or a diagnosis of candida overgrowth or small intestinal bacterial overgrowth (SIBO).

But you can heal leaky gut by decreasing inflammation, healing the mucosal lining of your gut, and increasing your ratio of beneficial to pathogenic microbes and your microbial diversity (meaning you have more different kinds of microbes). One of the best ways to increase the variety of good microbes in your gut is to increase the variety of foods you eat. Eat lots of different fruits and vegetables, according to what's in season. Vary your protein, including multiple sources of animal and plant protein (and dairy if you tolerate it). Take in a variety of different kinds of fats. Use a range of herbs and spices, which contain polyphenols that nourish the microbiome.

Fiber is another important dietary focus for a healthier microbiome and better blood sugar balance because the beneficial bacteria in your microbiome feed on fiber. The best way to get that fiber may be through vegetables, fruits, and nuts. In one study comparing groups eating a high-fiber diet based on fruits, vegetables, and nuts with another group eating a high-fiber diet based on grains and beans, the vegetable/fruit/nut group fared best.[9]

Interestingly, exercise also plays a major role in microbiome diversity. Exercise has been shown to improve the abundance of healthy bacteria in the gut, boost immunity, improve gut barrier function, and improve functional metabolic capacity.[10]

## Biohacking Your Gut Health

The best way to get a better sense of what's going on in your microbiome is to get it tested. I don't recommend bothering with stool tests you can order online, which don't yield much useful information. In order to get the level of analysis described below, I recommend visiting a functional medicine doctor who can order a clinical-grade stool test. That said, I want to add a disclaimer: there is a lot of controversy over whether functional stool studies are useful for optimizing gut health. When I describe these tests, I am writing from personal clinical experience and how I look at these markers and what I do about them. There are many doctors and scientists who don't believe we have enough evidence to recommend this kind of testing or the interventions I describe. But I have identified patients with bleeding polyps, inflammatory bowel diseases, compromised gut barrier function, intestinal infections, and enzyme insufficiency using these tests, so I believe they are useful. And, I've used these tests to optimize gut health by responding to this information. Even if you don't plan to get these tests, this list will tell you how you can improve different aspects of your microbiome health:

- **COMMENSAL RELATIVE ABUNDANCE.** This is a test to see how abundant the microbes that benefit your health (such as those supporting your immune system) are in your system, compared to those that have a more negative (inflammatory) effect. For low beneficial microbes, you can take prebiotics and probiotics to boost them. If they're high, your doctor should check for hydrogen or methane small intestinal bacterial overgrowth (SIBO).

- **SIGA.** This antibody is produced across mucosal surfaces and is the first line of defense in protecting your gut lining. Too much could be a sign of an overactive immune system due to infection, allergies, or autoimmunity. If no infections are found, I would recommend doing an elimination diet for a month to look for food sensitivities that might be compromising immunity. For that I recommend supplementing. Too little could be a sign of an underactive immune system, and in this case I would recommend supplementing with colostrum,

L-glutamine, prebiotics, and probiotics like *Saccharomyces boulardii*, a beneficial yeast.

- **SCFAS (SHORT-CHAIN FATTY ACIDS).** These are products produced by beneficial bacteria—mainly butyrate, acetate, and propionate—that help to maintain the gut lining and reduce inflammation in the digestive tract. If they are low, you need more fiber, prebiotics, polyphenols, and resistant starch, all of which nourish the beneficial bacteria that produce SCFAs. Ghee contains butyrate, so if you aren't sensitive to dairy, this is a good fat to use.

- **ELEVATED PRODUCTS OF PROTEIN BREAKDOWN OR UNDIGESTED FOOD FOUND IN STOOL.** This means either you're eating too much protein or you have insufficient enzymes to properly digest your food. When I see this, I advise chewing food more thoroughly and supplementing with digestive enzymes. Consider following a naturopathic hydrochloric acid (HCL) protocol to identify if you have low stomach acid and need to supplement with betaine HCL.

- **PANCREATIC ELASTASE.** This is an enzyme produced by the pancreas that helps to break down the food you eat and is an essential part of digestion. If it's low, you may benefit from taking digestive enzymes.

- **YEAST OVERGROWTH.** If you have an overgrowth of yeast, specifically various species of candida, it's a good idea to cut down on sugar (candida thrives on sugar). In severe cases, you can get a prescription for antifungals, but you can try treating mild cases with garlic, berberine, caprylic acid, and oregano oil.

- **BETA-GLUCURONIDASE.** This enzyme, if elevated, can lead to estrogen dominance, as it inhibits the excretion of estrogen.[11] It's often high in people who eat a high-fat, high-protein, low-fiber diet. Use calcium D-glucarate to inhibit the action of this enzyme.

- **FECAL FAT.** If you have fat in your stool, you may need more bile acids. Herbs like dandelion root, milk thistle seed, ginger, taurine, vitamin C, licorice, turmeric, and phosphatidylcholine to support gallbladder function can also help.

- **LOW AKKERMANSIA.** *Akkermansia* is a type of gut microbe that degrades mucus in the gastrointestinal tract. If it's low, you need more polyphenols to boost it. *Akkermansia* thrives on polyphenols, which you can get from eating more dark-colored berries, like blueberries; more herbs and spices; cocoa powder; and vegetables. Coffee and tea also contain polyphenols.

- **PARASITES.** If you have parasites in your gut, see a functional medical professional about appropriate treatment. You'll need to go on either an herbal or a prescription regimen to eliminate them.

- **OXALOBACTER FORMIGENES.** This is a beneficial gut bacterium that helps reduce the risk of calcium oxalate kidney stones.[12] People with urinary oxalates tend to have low levels of *O. formigenes,* and this increases their kidney stone risk. If your *O. formigenes* is low and you get kidney stones, you may want to avoid high-oxalate foods (like spinach and black tea.)[13]

- **H. PYLORI.** This is the bacterium that is associated with stomach ulcers and risk for developing stomach cancer. If it's elevated, I recommend herbal or prescription antimicrobial therapy. Mastic gum is a good supplement to take for *H. pylori*. You will want to see a good functional doctor to treat this.

- ZONULIN. This protein regulates intestinal permeability, and if it's high, that indicates that the mucosal barrier integrity has been compromised—i.e., you have a leaky gut. A 5R Program as described below would be helpful here. Support GI mucosal integrity through dietary intake of bone broth, gelatin, collagen, and fermented foods.

- EOSINOPHILIC PROTEIN X. This protein is a marker of eosinophil activation and degranulation, which can cause inflammatory allergic reactions. If it tests high, it could be due to a parasite, food allergies, or inflammatory bowel diseases like Crohn's or ulcerative colitis.

- CALPROTECTIN. This protein binds with calcium and zinc and is a marker of gut inflammation.[14] If you have high levels, you should get a professional workup for inflammatory bowel disease. I also would recommend starting an autoimmune paleo diet (e.g., the book *The Wahls Protocol* is excellent), which eliminates wheat, dairy, grains, and legumes/lectins from your diet. It can also be helpful to take anti-inflammatory supplements, especially boswellia and curcumin.

- OCCULT BLOOD. This is blood in the stool that you can't see, so you wouldn't notice it without a test. It indicates that you have some bleeding in your digestive tract, possibly caused by hemorrhoids, a colon polyp, or an arteriovenous malformation. If you get this result, you should get checked for hemorrhoids and consider getting a repeat test to verify, and/or getting a colonoscopy to check for polyps or cancer.

I've given you a lot of remedies for various lab results overall, but for healing and optimizing gut function, you should work with a functional doctor who can administer a 5R program for gut healing and optimization. This program includes (1) removing anything that is causing problems (e.g., allergenic foods, pathogenic bacteria, yeast, or parasites), (2) replacing anything that is missing (e.g., HCL, enzymes, bile acids, etc.), (3) repairing the gut barrier (e.g., using products like liquid fulvic and humic acids, L-glutamine, licorice, aloe vera, slippery elm, marshmallow, and cat's claw) and going on a GAPS or specific carbohydrate diet designed for gut healing, (4) reinoculating using pre-biotics, polyphenols, and probiotic foods and supplements, and (5) re-laxing by reducing stress, which plays a role in impaired digestion.

After all this technical information, I want to remind you that most of what influences how you feel, the state of your blood sugar and in-sulin, and the health of your microbiome is the food you eat. I find it helps to have some basic rules or boundaries around food and eating that keep me on track, so I eat in a way that is most likely to make me feel good, keep my blood sugar in balance, and feed the beneficial bacteria in my microbiome. Everyone will have their own guidelines for how to eat and live. Yours may not be the same as mine, but I rec-ommend making a list that fits your needs. This is my simple list—let it inspire you to make your own:

- EAT MINDFULLY. I plan my meals purposefully and pay attention to what I'm eating.
- SNACK MINDFULLY. I try not to snack much, but when I really need to, I plan it with as much purpose and eat it with as much attention as I do a full meal.
- SIT DOWN TO EAT. If I'm going to eat, I commit and sit down.
- EAT HIGH-QUALITY FOOD. You want nutrient density over food quantity. Choose the highest-quality food you can afford. If you're going to eat dessert, make sure it's really worth it, or make your own from scratch.
- SHOP LIKE A CHEF AND KNOW YOUR SOURCES. I try to think like a chef when I buy food, and buy local and meet the farmers who grow my food whenever possible.
- NO AIRPLANE FOOD. Nothing makes jet lag worse than eating crappy airplane food. Bring your own food on airplanes. My favorite things

are nuts and seeds, dark chocolate, hard-boiled eggs, flax crackers and hummus, and kale chips.

o   **NO FAST FOOD**. It's not actually food! Once you cut it out, you won't miss it.

I hope this inspires you to create a diet you love that is customized to your preferences, sensitivities, blood sugar variability, and microbiome. This is the ultimate way to improve your metabolic health and the way you feel overall.

---

### MICROBIOME BIOHACKS IN THIS CHAPTER

- Get a gut health test from a functional doctor to assess your microbiome health, so you can address any issues you discover.

- If you have serious gut issues, find a doctor who can work with you on a 5R program.

- Live a gut-healthy lifestyle by eating mindfully, choosing high-quality food, avoiding junk, and shopping from local natural food and farmers markets.

- Eat a wide variety of foods to improve your microbiome diversity.

- Assess yourself for signs of intestinal permeability, a.k.a. leaky gut.

# CHAPTER 9

# Biohacking
# Energy Metabolism

Everyone can perform magic, everyone can reach his goals, if he is able to think, if he is able to wait, if he is able to fast.

—Hermann Hesse

Metabolic flexibility is the ability to efficiently adapt metabolism to different fuel sources—i.e., being able to switch from burning glucose (from carbs and protein) to burning ketones (from fat). When you are metabolically flexible, you can easily toggle between these sources, which blunts blood sugar spikes and helps maintain a low insulin state in the body. This used to be necessary in times of food scarcity—when carbs were available, such as in the summer, we would feast on them. When they weren't, such as in the winter, when we might only find animals to eat—or nothing to eat—our bodies had to learn to switch to using dietary fat, or our own fat stores, for fuel.

Because we evolved like this, metabolic flexibility should come naturally. Say you had to run for an hour, using about seven hundred calories, four hours after a meal. First you would burn the sugar in your blood from your last meal, then you would tap into your glycogen (the stored fuel in the liver and muscles). After that, if you're going to keep going, your body must switch to burning fat for fuel, because it's the only fuel you have left. If your body doesn't know how to do this, you won't be able to keep going and you will "bonk," as athletes call it, meaning you'll suddenly be overwhelmed with fatigue and weakness.

I'll never forget the time I helped a colleague work on becoming more metabolically flexible with mild fasting and intermittent ketosis, which we tracked with a glucose monitor and ketone monitor. A few weeks into our work together, she decided to participate in a triathlon that she hadn't fully trained for. One of her friends had been training for weeks on a high-carb diet using all sorts of sugar-based gels to power her activity. When competition day came along, my colleague ended up finishing the race ahead of her friend, who didn't finish the race because she "bonked" when she ran out of carbs for fuel. My colleague was able to finish the race (untrained) because she was so metabolically flexible that she could tap into fat for fuel when she ran out of glycogen.

A great way to biohack metabolic flexibility is to purposefully reduce carbohydrate intake. You can do this by eating very low-carb, like a ketogenic diet, or eating nothing at all for a while, i.e., fasting. This

## GRAZING HINDERS METABOLIC FLEXIBILITY

A common barrier to metabolic flexibility is simply eating too often. Between 2009 and 2014, according to the CDC's National Health and Nutrition Examination Survey data, Americans reported about five eating episodes a day, with the dinner meal and the after-dinner snack being the most common meals reported, contributing to 45 percent of daily energy intake. The average dinner time is 6:24 P.M., ending at 8:18 p.m.[1] This stores enough glycogen in the liver to fuel the body for ten to fourteen hours (assuming no exercise). Eating this often and late won't allow your body to use up your glycogen. I call this clogging the glycogen sink. It's highly beneficial to health to drain that glycogen sink occasionally by going for longer periods without eating. This flips the metabolic switch to burning fat for fuel, and that helps your body become more metabolically flexible. If you don't drain the glycogen sink overnight, you won't go into fat burning while sleeping. If you've already got plenty of stored glycogen, whatever fuel you eat from dinner and later gets stored as extra fat.[2]

gives your body the opportunity to practice switching—when it runs out of glucose and glycogen, which it will quickly do if you aren't eating carbs, it gets forced to search for alternative fuel. You are essentially making your body "practice" fuel switching, something it may not otherwise ever get the chance to do since people generally eat so often and eat so many carbs.

Or, in the case of people who almost always eat a low-carb diet and have lost the metabolic flexibility they need to easily switch to sugar burning, you can help your body practice fuel switching by cycling through periods where you eat more carbs. The more you force your body to switch fuel supplies, the better your body gets at doing it.

## How to Build Metabolic Flexibility

There are multiple ways to biohack your metabolic flexibility, and most of them have to do with varying when you eat, when you move, and what you do. Just as hormesis builds resilience, toggling between stressor and recovery, variation builds resilience, and metabolic flexibility is metabolic resilience. Here are some ways to do this.

- **VARIABLE EXERCISE.** Train different muscle fiber systems so your body learns to adapt to different demands. Exercise can have a significant effect on how the body handles glucose. For example, moderate-intensity aerobic exercise improves insulin sensitivity and increases the efficiency of glucose use. HIIT improves the number and function of mitochondria available to burn carbs and efficiently depletes glycogen stores. Weight lifting makes a bigger sink for glycogen to go into by increasing muscle (and therefore increasing glycogen use).[3]

- **FOLLOWING NATURE'S LEAD.** A natural way to live in harmony with the seasons and also increase metabolic flexibility is to imitate how humans used to live. In the winter, people likely slept more because it was darker for longer, ate fewer carbs because they were less available, and didn't move as much because of the weather. In summer, they probably moved more because it was nice outside and ate more carbs because they were available. You could mimic this by sleeping more, eating a lower-carbohydrate diet, and focusing on weight lifting in the winter, and getting more active, sleeping less, eating a higher-carb diet, and getting more outdoor exercise in the summer.

• **NUTRITIONAL PERIODIZATION, OR CARB CYCLING.** Vary your macronutrient ratios to suit your metabolic needs, current lifestyle, and stress levels. For instance, eat a diet with a moderate carb level when you are stressed, to send signals to your body that you are safe, and eat a higher-fat, lower-carb diet when you are feeling strong and relaxed, to hone your metabolic flexibility. This enables your body to become or stay flexible in the context of different challenges. You can also develop a regular schedule for cycling your macros (protein, carbs, fat) and calorie goals to intentionally train your body to become more metabolically flexible.

• **FASTING.** Intermittent fasting depletes glycogen stores and trains your body to tap into its fat stores once you get into ketosis, flipping the metabolic switch and increasing autophagy (the body getting rid of dead and damaged cells) and mitophagy (the body getting rid of dysfunctional mitochondria). For some people, fasting by taking in fewer than 500 calories (or no calories) once or twice a week may be an easier weight loss strategy than continuous caloric restriction. Both regimens achieve a calorie deficit. The main difference between fasting and caloric restriction is the longer you go without food, the more likely you are to flip the metabolic switch and produce ketones, which have their own positive effects on mitochondrial, muscle, and brain health.

- **PERIODIC CALORIE RESTRICTION.** Given how many women struggle with weight loss, eating disorders, and chronic stress, I'm not advocating a diet here. Chronic calorie restriction (dieting) isn't the path to a high-quality life, in my opinion. It's like chronic stress—there's no recovery time. We were designed to occasionally limit our calories in cycles. A constant diet that is always the same also doesn't match the natural way humans have eaten. Until very recently in the scope of human existence, humans have had to eat what they could find and what was in season, and that was always changing. But eating a lower-calorie diet a few days a week and a higher-calorie diet a few days a week can teach your body to become metabolically flexible. Continuous calorie restriction tends to lower the basal metabolic rate, but undulating your calories day-to-day can teach the body to adapt to more or less food and make cells more metabolically flexible in the process.

## Fasting: A Powerful Way to Become Metabolically Flexible

The word *fasting* tends to trigger some strong opinions. Some people love fasting, some people hate it, and some people are curious but afraid to try it. But as trendy as it might seem, intermittent fasting has ancient roots. It's the way humans evolved to interact with food. The only reason it *feels* new is because we're used to eating so much and so often.

For most of human existence, endurance exercise and fasting were signals to the body to promote cellular resilience by performing functions like cellular housecleaning to throw out dysfunctional proteins and mitochondria, and increasing neurogenesis to resist brain cell degeneration and increase our ability to solve problems (like finding more food or getting out of danger). The adaptation of flipping a switch from carb burning to fat mobilization and ketosis enabled our ancestors to tolerate food deprivation, which provided a massive survival advantage.

We are still built to receive those signals—it's just that most people don't do endurance exercise and don't go for very long without food anymore. By not moving and constantly eating, we are missing a great opportunity to increase health and expand healthspan.[4] The natural rhythm of life is to feast and fast. There are times to feast, like for special occasions, and there are times when going without food is exactly what the body needs.

Fasting feels uncomfortable to many people, mostly because they aren't used to it and aren't metabolically flexible, so their bodies have trouble flipping the switch from sugar burning to fat burning. After reading Dr. Jason Fung's *The Complete Guide to Fasting*, I used fasting to help heal my insulin resistance. It does not work for everyone (the naturally lean out there seem to be particularly resistant to fasting), but it can make a huge difference in your health if you have metabolic dysfunction. Does this mean you have to fast if you want to heal your metabolism problems? No! Some people make fantastic progress using the mainstays of calorie restriction, aerobic exercise, and weight training to achieve their health and fitness goals. But, a lot of people have failed on these traditional paths and found fasting to work for them in combination with a healthy diet and exercise regimen.

It's safe as long as you maintain healthy body fat and muscle mass levels and a healthy relationship with food. It helps your brain work better, boosting BDNF and improving mental clarity and concentration. It improves wound healing. It increases fertility in people with obesity. It can reduce cholesterol levels, blood pressure, triglycerides, inflammation, and oxidative stress.[5] It does all this because it reduces the burden on the mitochondria and the microbes in your gut, so they don't have to work so hard. For all these reasons and more, we should stop vilifying fasting and recognize that it is a tool appropriate for some (not all) people to improve metabolism.

I lowered my fasting glucose using fasting, and many of my patients have experienced similar results. I've seen fasting reverse SIBO. I've had friends with inflammatory bowel diseases go into remission with regular intermittent fasting. It also promotes detoxification by upregulating endogenous antioxidant systems in the liver (meaning it helps your liver produce its own antioxidants, which can help to combat free radicals and reduce inflammation). It reduces weight by enabling a caloric deficit. It increases ketones, which can help improve focus and boost brain health. In animal studies, fasting lengthened the lifespan of animals, and fasting may increase longevity in humans as well.[6]

Body fat, at its core, is stored energy for us to "eat" when there is no food. When we fast, we "eat" our own fat (this, in essence, is ketosis). The body could make energy from food, but it can also make energy from stored fuel. A 140-pound woman with 23 percent body fat has 32.2 pounds of stored fuel in the form of fat, and that equates to 112,000 calories' worth of fuel. That's enough to last more than a month without food—not that you should (there are all sorts of things that go wrong when people fast for weeks and I would never recommend this without supervision), but it's interesting to consider how much stored fuel we are carrying around on our bodies.

Fasting is particularly helpful for people with insulin resistance, prediabetes, or diabetes; people who are sedentary; and people who are overweight or obese. It can also be a useful tool for healthy people who want to train their bodies and their minds to handle the challenge of going without food. Other people do it for its longevity benefits, such as inducing autophagy and promoting brain health. It can also help with mental fitness. In my personal experience, longer fasts were a major catalyst for spiritual growth, but my current fasting regimen mostly consists of twelve- to fourteen-hour fasts, with the occasional twenty-four-hour fast.

## Who Shouldn't Fast

Before I get into the details of how to fast, a disclaimer: if you are young (in your twenties) and healthy, you probably don't need to do a lot of fasting, if any. Being young doesn't bar you from fasting, and I've found that plenty of young men love it, but young women who are fertile and healthy (without problems like PCOS) may not need to fast more than twelve hours. They can achieve ketosis through exercise and carb cycling. Fasting can be too stressful because they're already metabolically flexible. It's important to develop healthy eating habits when you are young rather than emphasize fasting.

Athletes also have to be careful. Female athletes are more likely to experience hormone dysfunction if they fast (or just undereat) while engaging in strenuous activity. For most athletes, especially those who are young women, the priority should be to make sure you are eating the right foods and not limiting your calories. I dig into Relative Energy Deficiency of Sport in chapter 12, which is a health condition not to take lightly.

The cool thing about exercise is that it offers a lot of the same cellular housecleaning benefits as fasting, which is why sedentary people may be better candidates for fasting than athletes. Fasting becomes more important as we age and lose that metabolic flexibility. Remember, there's a difference in the biological imperatives of men and women, and there is also a difference in the biological imperatives of young and old. Young people are in a growth state. Data suggests that calorie restriction and intermittent fasting can compromise certain immune responses in juveniles but can enhance immune function in adults. As individuals get older, into their thirties, forties, fifties, and beyond, fasting becomes much more useful. Even then, remember to pay attention to how your body responds. It will tell you if what you're doing is working or if you should stop.

Other situations where people should not fast: if they have excessively low body fat, are pregnant or breastfeeding, are new to health and wellness, or have a sleep disorder. It's also so important to understand that fasting can exacerbate a current or past eating disorder. *If you have a history of eating disorders, I recommend skipping this section altogether.* The benefits are not worth the risks, in my opinion.

If you're diabetic, I recommend consulting with your doctor before you begin a fasting regimen because it can impact your need for insulin and other medications and you may end up needing to lower your doses.

Finally, if you are dealing with a lot of stress and have signs of hormonal dysfunction like thyroid problems or low cortisol, your focus should not be on fasting. It should be on recovery from stress, which can take six to nine months. I can't emphasize this enough. After a period of extreme stress during the COVID-19 pandemic, I struggled with fasting and found I just couldn't do it anymore. My body was telling me it wasn't the right time to pile stressors on top of stressors. When you are in a state of chronic stress, regular meal timing is key, including protein first thing in the morning, sufficient carbs at each meal (aiming for no less than 100 grams of carbs a day), and potentially a small snack before bed. While recovering from chronic stress, focus on restorative activities like meditation, yoga, plenty of sleep, and time in nature and with your community, not metabolic stressors like fasting or ketosis. Okay, disclaimers over.

## How to Begin Fasting

When I first started fasting, I found it challenging. I couldn't do it because I wasn't very metabolically flexible. People who start fasting and feel sick, faint, or nauseous are showing signs that they are not metabolically flexible enough to be fasting. When people "fail" their

> ## ISN'T FASTING STARVATION?
>
> A lot of people object to fasting, thinking it's the same as starving, but fasting is completely different from starvation in one crucial way: choice. When you fast, you have a choice to resume eating normally. People who live during famines or who have eating disorders are unable to maintain a healthy caloric balance because it is out of their control. In the case of anorexia nervosa or anorexia athletica, individuals starve themselves or exercise themselves to the point of having very low body weight and body fat and have a difficult time maintaining a healthy body composition because of their condition. With healthy fasting, you don't get to that point. You do it long enough to benefit but not so long that you cause harm.

fast and give up, it is usually that they are metabolically inflexible.[7] This population should first focus on training their bodies to drop into ketosis by becoming fat adapted through a ketogenic diet (page 163) to flip the metabolic switch before starting a fast.

To get into nutritional ketosis to develop your metabolic flexibility, track how many carbs you eat. Nutritional ketosis occurs when eating fewer than 50 grams of net carbohydrates a day. It usually takes two to four days to increase ketones in the blood. The goal here is getting "fat adapted," meaning you have gotten your metabolic machinery capable of burning fat effectively as fuel. This can take between one and three months (and sometimes even longer). Nutritional ketosis offers a lot of the same benefits as fasting, such as appetite reduction, carbohydrate craving reduction, weight loss, visceral fat loss, lowered triglycerides, increased HDL (good cholesterol), lowered blood sugar, and lowered blood pressure.[8]

This gradual progression into fasting will be a lot more comfortable after a period of ketosis, but it can still take your body some time to get used to fasting. The first few tries might feel difficult. Be prepared, not discouraged. It really does get easier. Fasting is no different from any other life skill: practice and support are essential to performing it well, but as with any change, our bodies prefer to adapt slowly.

To ease into fasting, follow these steps in order and take as long as feels comfortable at each interval before moving on (and know you can go back a step or can stop at any time). Here is your progression:

## STEP ONE: START WITH REGULAR MEALTIMES
## AND CUTTING OUT SNACKING

Get on a consistent meal schedule. Consistent meal timing can help reduce leptin, a hormone that produces hunger signals, and insulin resistance. It can also normalize stress hormones. Starting your day with a protein-rich breakfast can also help with leptin sensitivity. Eating regular meals without snacking takes practice, but snacking is often just a habit. So many people just snack all day long, and it makes it so much harder to fast. I'm not saying you can't ever snack, but I am saying that most people are snacking much more than they should, causing excess insulin output. This makes it much harder to fast. Try to avoid eating in front of your computer, in the car, in front of the TV, at the movies, or in class.

## STEP TWO: SWITCH TO A WHOLE-FOOD DIET

The transition to fasting will feel much more natural when you first eliminate fast food and packaged, processed food. Eating whole foods and eliminating processed foods will increase your metabolic flexibility. Your body won't have that desperate addictive hunger around processed foods. Set yourself free from that first, and not eating for short periods will feel so much easier. Quitting sugar for a month can be especially helpful for breaking sugar cravings.

### STEP THREE: BEGIN CUTTING CARBS OR IMPLEMENT
### A KETOGENIC DIET FOR A MONTH

Helping your body get used to less glucose and nudging it toward fat burning can make fasting much easier. You can start by gradually cutting back on carbs. This is the real secret: the easiest way to become fat adapted is to eat a ketogenic diet that is high in fat and contains fewer than 50 grams of carbs per day.[9] The carbohydrate limit any individual person needs to get into ketosis varies, which is why testing ketones is useful. Ketosis reduces insulin signaling and gets your body accustomed to surviving without glucose, refining your metabolic flexibility so fasting doesn't feel as extreme. It also helps decrease appetite and increase satisfaction on less food, and it can help with weight loss without suppressing metabolic rate.[10] You know you are fat adapted when you aren't hungry all the time, you have fewer carbohydrate cravings, you don't need to snack constantly, you can skip a meal here and there without getting hangry, and you have fewer mood swings and energy swings after meals.

### STEP FOUR: STOP EATING BETWEEN SIX AND EIGHT P.M.

This will help you sync up to your natural circadian rhythm. Avoid late-night snacking. This can help your body align with the natural light and dark cycles and may reduce your blood sugar the next day. It will also make overnight fasting feel easier.

### STEP FIVE: START WITH A TWELVE-HOUR FAST

This is by far the most gradual way to begin an intermittent fast with the least amount of pain, and it's the maximum amount of time women who are athletes should be fasting. If you finish eating at eight P.M., you don't eat again until eight A.M. You might already be doing this, but if you aren't, you might have to change some habits. I am personally doing this more often than not, and sometimes I'll do a fourteen-hour fast. This is where most young and healthy people should stay.

### STEP SIX: INCREASE TO A 14:10 FAST

The next step is to fast for fourteen hours, with a ten-hour eating window. This is a good place for young, healthy, less active women who aren't athletes to settle. If you stop eating at eight P.M., you would not have breakfast until ten A.M. Gradually increasing to fourteen hours shouldn't hurt most people, but you really should keep an eye on your

---

### HOW TO "DO KETO"

There are many different ways to do a ketogenic diet, and a lot of people have written whole books on this subject that you can check out. Anyone can eat in a keto pattern by tracking macros and consuming a high-healthy-fat, moderate-protein, very low-carb diet. To see if it's working, you can test your ketones. If you want macro targets to shoot for, or options, here are some basic types of ketogenic diets to choose from, but again, I encourage you to do some research to find a keto plan that works for you, if you aren't comfortable figuring it out for yourself.

- **STANDARD KETOGENIC DIET (SKD).** This typically consists of 70 percent fat, 20 percent protein, and 10 percent carbs.

- **CYCLICAL KETOGENIC DIET (CKD).** This diet alternates periods of higher-carb eating with a standard ketogenic diet, such as five ketogenic days followed by two normal-carb days. That doesn't mean refined carbs, though. Emphasize whole-food carbs like root vegetables and fruit.

- **TARGETED KETOGENIC DIET (TKD).** This diet allows you to add more carbs on workout days.

- **HIGH-PROTEIN KETOGENIC DIET.** This version is similar to standard keto but includes more protein. Your macros would look more like 60 percent fat, 35 percent protein, and 5 percent carbs.

## TOOLS FOR A KETOGENIC DIET:

- **MAGNESIUM AND ELECTROLYTES.** Your body needs more of these because you are often shedding water, which can contribute to dehydration and muscle cramping.

- **DIGESTIVE ENZYMES, BETAINE HCL, AND BILE ACIDS** can help you digest extra fat. I have protocols for these on my website. Spices such as ginger, turmeric, fresh black pepper, and chili powder can also help stimulate bile flow.

- **GREEN POWDERS.** Ideally, you will get your veggies from food, but for people who aren't accustomed to eating a lot of veggies, I do recommend these in a pinch. They are an easy way to digest green vegetables.

- **KETONE MONITORS.** You can buy ketone monitors over the counter. Look for the ones that use blood, not urine—they are more accurate. You do have to stick your finger periodically but the information is worth it, in my opinion. There are also breath-testing tools for checking whether you are burning sugar or ketones, but I have not personally determined their accuracy. Blood ketones are best measured on a fasting stomach and in the morning:

  Below 0.5 mmol/L is not considered ketosis.

  0.5–1.5 mmol/L is light nutritional ketosis, which might have a positive effect on your weight.

  1.5–3 mmol/L is optimal ketosis, and this is considered the best spot for maximum weight loss. 1.5–3 is easier to achieve if you're pairing fasting with ketogenic dieting, especially if you are obese.

  Going above 3 mmol/L is totally unnecessary and won't help you get better results.

body fat. A study showed that when overweight individuals did twelve-to-fourteen-hour fasts for sixteen weeks, they had lowered body weight and better sleep, and this persisted for a year.[11] You may never want or need to go beyond fourteen hours, but if you are sedentary, it's especially important not to eat after dinner.

### EXERCISE DURING FASTING

There are conflicting opinions about whether to exercise before or after eating. Exercising in a fasted state (such as first thing in the morning before breakfast) makes exercise harder. It's kind of like exercising with a weighted vest. I know many men who feel great exercising fasted, which is a sign that they can handle it. Men seem to tolerate exercising and fasting better than women, but I wouldn't make it a habit for anyone not in strong metabolic and mental health.

I don't recommend combining strenuous exercise and fasting for women. If you are a female athlete, you need a small 150-calorie meal before working out, especially before morning workouts, to bring your blood sugar up enough! Fasting offers a lot of the same effects as exercise, so you don't need both. Fasted cardio or weight lifting in women elevates cortisol and will increase body fat storage. During intermittent fasting you can do gentle yoga and walks, but save strenuous exercise for midday, when you're eating, versus when you're fasted.

### STEP SEVEN: INCREASE TO A 16:8 FAST

A 16:8 fast might look like stopping eating at six P.M. and then not eating the next day until ten A.M. It is likely to have the greatest benefits in individuals with insulin resistance and impaired blood sugar or fat metabolism.[12] This strategy may help menopausal women lose fat while preserving lean body mass.[13] It's a great ratio for people who aren't exercising, and if you have obesity or need to lose weight, this ratio can help you get to your goal weight and stabilize your blood sugar. Many people find a 16:8 fast helps reduce appetite in the morning and increase fullness in the evening, which can aid in weight loss. But you can take anything too far too fast—don't jump into this right away. If this works and feels great, you may even want to progress to longer fasts.

## WHAT TO EXPECT DURING YOUR FIRST FAST

During your first extended fast, when you go longer than you usually do without eating—for many people, it's that 16:8 fast that starts to feel difficult—you might feel hunger pangs, mild abdominal discomfort, or weakness. You might feel light-headed, you could feel some cramps, you could feel dehydrated, you might not sleep well, and you might lose some weight. Most of these symptoms can be remedied with electrolytes, focusing on fat adaptation first (eating a ketogenic diet before fasting for this long), going slowly and gradually into this level of fasting, and experience. The more your body gets used to fasting, the fewer symptoms you will have.

If you are mildly stressed but you still want to try it, be extra gentle. Two weeks of intermittent fasting has been shown not to raise cortisol levels, although this could depend on how stressed you actually are.

There are so many rewards to fasting! It builds willpower, discipline, patience, flexibility, resilience, and adaptability. It makes your skin radiant, it's simple, it's free, and you'll save money because you're eating less. It's convenient because you don't have to keep stopping what you're doing to eat. It makes food taste better, heightening your senses, especially your taste buds.[14]

Some people find that fasting helps them connect to their purpose in life and their spirituality. For a lot of people, regular exercise is more intimidating than occasional fasting, so learning how to fast is easier to tackle psychologically. If you're an avid exerciser or athlete, you really don't need to fast as much, but if you aren't active and are looking to improve your metabolic health (e.g. especially if you're insulin resistant, prediabetic, have metabolic syndrome, or are overweight or obese) fasting may be worth trying. It doesn't work for everyone, but it can be a great tool in your biohacking toolbox.

## TIPS TO MAKE FASTING EASIER

Fasting takes some practice when you aren't used to going for long periods without eating. To help ease the transition, progress slowly. It can also help if you:

- **STAY HYDRATED.** This is my number one tip. If you don't hydrate, you'll feel sick, extra fatigued, or weak. Besides water, you can drink sparkling water, black coffee, or tea. Just don't use any added sugar. If you like to drink coffee or tea, just recognize that caffeine during fasting may help with fat burning, but it can also stress the body, so make sure you're having two to three cups of water between your cups of caffeine.

- **GET ENOUGH ELECTROLYTES.** Water follows salt. You may need to take a sugar-free electrolyte supplement or add a few pinches of salt to your water, to stay properly hydrated. Magnesium is great for people who get headaches when they start to fast. I skip most supplements on days that I am fasting, but I do like magnesium glycinate or threonate for headaches.

- **FASTING APPS AND A SMART SCALE.** There are great apps out there for fasting, along with scales that read more than just your weight—they scan you for body fat percentage, muscle mass, and other metrics. I have some product recommendations on my website.

- **KNOW WHEN TO QUIT.** If you feel faint or so unwell that you aren't able to function properly, please stop the fast and focus on building metabolic flexibility first, through a period of ketosis or cyclical ketosis.

## METABOLIC FLEXIBILITY BIOHACKS IN THIS CHAPTER

- Vary your habits, diet, exercise, and eating periods to mimic natural cycles and improve your metabolic flexibility.

- Assess your stress level and health to determine whether you are fit for fasting.

- Warm up to fasting by trying a ketogenic diet.

- Progress slowly to fasting. Start by getting in the habit of having regular mealtimes, not snacking, and eating a whole-food diet.

- Begin cutting carbs or do a ketogenic diet for one month.

- Switch your largest meal to lunch and stop eating by six to eight p.m.

- Start with a twelve to fourteen hour overnight fast.

- Don't do strenuous exercise without eating.

- Experiment with longer fasting techniques if they appeal to you.

- Be cautious if you plan to fast for more than three days, as this can cause health problems.

- Try a ketone monitoring system to test whether you are in ketosis.

- Add electrolytes and magnesium supplements to support your fast.

- Try using a fasting app.

- Ease back into eating with small digestible meals.

# PART IV

# USING YOUR BATTERIES

# CHAPTER 10

# Stress Drains Your Batteries

Focusing on health, I expressly reject the implicit assumption that stressors are inherently pathogenic. Their health consequences can only be understood if we understand the coping process.

—Aaron Antonovsky

Life is stressful, and that's normal. Life has always been stressful. The stressors are different than they once were, but we were built to handle the ups and downs of stress—emergency, recovery, emergency, recovery. If we didn't have the capacity to endure stress, we wouldn't have survived as a species.

Stress is not inherently bad (remember hormesis). It has been said that intelligence is the ability to adapt to change and I believe health is the ability to adapt in the face of adversity. Health is about resilience, and the way the body learns to adapt and be resilient is through experiencing challenges and overcoming them to become stronger.

Recovering from stress is essential for maintaining health and extending healthspan. But, achieving meaningful recovery can be a real challenge in this modern world. The problem is chronic, unrelenting stress that we can't escape because it continues to pile up every day.

Some doctors will tell you that chronic stress is the culprit behind most chronic disease; however, few can offer actionable ways to help you master your stress response. One important reason is that people often overlook, or don't know about, the chronic stressors that we don't even realize are there. This will make sense if we first look at how stress works.

## Understanding the Subtleties of the Stress Response

Acute stressors—such as an illness or injury or a stressful life event like a move, a divorce, or even something that's positive, like a marriage, having a baby, or getting a promotion—trigger the sympathetic nervous system, also known as our "fight or flight" mode. The acute stress response is adaptive and is designed to keep you alive. It initiates the release of stress hormones, like cortisol, so you can defend yourself. It increases neural plasticity in your brain so you can learn. It disrupts your circadian rhythm to make you adaptable to long nights or early mornings. It increases inflammation to protect you from germs. It resists insulin so more glucose goes to your brain. It increases motivation so you won't hesitate to act in the face of danger. It also shuts down functions that are secondary to immediate survival, like digestion and fertility, diverting resources to muscles and the brain. The body assumes that when you are fighting or fleeing for your life, you're not also going to be eating dinner or having sex.

The parasympathetic nervous system, which is traditionally associated with recovery after stress, also contributes to survival under stress. In the event we are overwhelmed with danger and cannot escape, the dorsal arm of the parasympathetic nervous system (PNS) will cause us to shut down and freeze. The PNS response helps to explain why, for example, when a woman is attacked (or sexually assaulted), she may freeze and not be able to fight back. Her nervous system is trying to protect her when there aren't better options for evading an attacker.

On the other hand, the ventral arm of the parasympathetic nervous system that takes over when we feel safe. This arm is the social engagement system that helps us recover from the acute stress. It's activated when we feel safe and are surrounded by people we love and trust. It allows for secondary functions like digestion and fertility to come back online. It is an elegant design that we have evolved to survive. Key takeaways are that the stress response is not a nuisance but rather is adaptive, helping you survive in times of acute, life-threatening danger, and recovery from stress helps you return to normal and thrive.

## LEVEL UP YOUR STRESS VOCABULARY

• **HOMEOSTASIS** is how your body maintains normal body temperature, electrolyte balance, blood sugar, blood pressure, and heart rate so you can survive and thrive.

• **ALLOSTASIS** is how the body adapts to psychological or environmental stress by changing internal parameters to maintain internal stability through change.

• **ALLOSTATIC LOAD** is the cumulative stress we experience. Imagine you are filling a cup with stress. The amount of stress in your cup is your allostatic load. The size of your cup is your allostatic capacity, and that depends on how much energy capacity you have. How full your cup is will depend on whether you have sufficiently recovered from your stressors.

• **ALLOSTATIC OVERLOAD** is what happens when the stress cup overflows and your bodily systems start to break down. This is how stress really begins to impact health.

Chronic stress is often less intense than acute stress, but if there isn't enough space to recover, you may find that you feel tightly wound and your body seems to be in a state of fear even where there is nothing to be afraid of. When your sympathetic nervous system is in overdrive, it becomes hypervigilant to any possible danger.

Chronic stress is damaging to the body and brain. It drains your organ reserves, makes you more vulnerable to illness, and restructures the brain, shrinking the hippocampus and reducing synaptic plasticity.[1]

Chronic stress also alters your circadian rhythm, increases inflammation and insulin resistance, and can depress your sense of motivation, pleasure, and reward.[2] All of this makes you less resilient and subject to allostatic overload, because your capacity decreases as your brain's threat system is constantly activated.[3] You may become more irritable, reactive, depressed, and more sensitive to minor threats. Your heart rate and blood pressure will be elevated too often. Your fasting blood sugar will stay higher. Over time, you can end up with heart disease, hypertension, or diabetes. This is how chronic stress leads to chronic disease.

## Hidden Sources of Stress

There are certain stealthy types of chronic stress that people often don't realize they have. Uncovering and resolving these hidden stressors can be important to lowering your overall stress burden and can free up a lot of extra energy.

The first type results from aspects of our environment that contribute to feeling unsafe. We can understand this phenomenon through a theory known as the Generalized Unsafety Theory of Stress, or GUTS.[4] GUTS offers an explanation of how a perceived feeling of unsafety in your internal or external environment contributes to your chronic stress level.

The second type of stress consists of childhood traumas, which includes extreme events known as adverse childhood experiences (ACEs). These events have significant ramifications on a person's health and are related to the development of chronic disease in adulthood.

## Feeling Unsafe: GUTS

The conventional theory of stress is that it is caused by punctuated stressors—this happens, then that happens, then this happens, and now you are stressed. The problem with this model is it ignores some of the low-level stressors around us that cause our nervous systems to become overactivated. Major life stressors will certainly influence your overall stress response. If you lose your job and your partner leaves you, of course you're going to experience significant stress. But remember that allostatic load is like a cup. If your cup is already nearly full due to low-grade stressors in your environment that you experience all the time, it won't take long for those punctuated stressors to cause allostatic overload.

According to Stephen Porges, PhD, founding director of the Traumatic Stress Research Consortium at Indiana University and professor of psychiatry at the University of North Carolina, we experience feelings of safety by default in groups of other people (because we evolved as pack animals).

But, according to GUTS, our isolating modern environment contributes to feelings of unsafety. From a GUTS perspective, our brain is always scanning our environment for threats and is only able to relax when we feel a sense of safety. A compromised social network—feeling lonely or isolated—puts us on high alert by default. We don't only experience stress in reaction to external challenges; we also experience stress due to a general feeling of unsafety from lack of connection to a community.

Compared to the lives our ancestors faced, our world is orders of magnitude safer than prehistoric societies, but in many ways, it is, or at least feels, less safe. Fear-based news media cycles, compromised health, financial or social insecurity, systemic racism and bias, a stressful work or home environment, isolation and loneliness, and less obvious unsafety signals than living in a dangerous, polluted, loud, or dark place can keep your brain from turning on the safety switch.

I had been living in San Francisco when I learned about GUTS. Consciously, I felt like I was leading a pretty good, safe existence, but I was waking up in the mornings unrested, and I didn't know why. I never felt fully relaxed. The reality is the discomforts of an urban environment—the noise, the pollution, not knowing my neighbors, being a woman living alone—were all very much present in the background. Although I didn't consciously focus on these environmental factors, learning about GUTS helped me realize how a subconscious sense of unsafety was filling my stress cup.

After I moved into a community living environment, I felt a lot better. But, it wasn't until I left the city and moved to Maui for a few months in early 2020 that I realized how much my previous life in San Francisco—with its environment noise pollution, wildfire smoke, and high crime rates—has been affecting my mental health. The chronic unsafety signaling was negatively impacting my nervous system.

According to GUTS, there are three highly prevalent conditions that keep us in a mode of feeling generally unsafe. They are:

1. **COMPROMISED BODY.** *If you have a reduced bodily capacity, even if you are not injured or ill, you will feel unsafe at an instinctual level. This could be from low fitness, obesity, reduced mobility, frailty, old age, or a combination of factors. If you aren't physically capable of running away or fighting, you may sense that you would have difficulty escaping physical danger. Your body knows that, so it feels unsafe.*

   *If you want to send a signal to your body that it's safe, you can work on building your strength and cardiorespiratory fitness, improving your mobility, getting to a healthy weight, and monitoring your heart rate and heart rate variability (I'll provide resources to tools I use on my website). These are all ways to turn on the "safety" switch because they help your body understand that you could more easily survive in an emergency. And that's also literally true. You never know when you might need to run fast to get away from something dangerous, whether that's jumping out of the way of a car, fleeing from someone chasing you, running from a wildfire sweeping into your neighborhood, or escaping a flood or some other natural disaster. Nobody is 100 percent perfectly fit and healthy in every way, and we all age. You can't reverse the clock, but this is one really important reason to prioritize improving your fitness.*

2. **COMPROMISED SOCIAL NETWORK.** *Our primary source of safety comes from being part of a cohesive social network. We used to live in tribes for protection, but now people have weaker or absent social ties. This, among other things, has contributed to the decline of the nuclear family and close-knit friend groups. We may not think we need these for survival anymore, but at an instinctual level, we still do. This is why our bodies interpret loneliness as danger.*

*You can think of loneliness as a primitive pain signal designed to bring you closer to your community—because being isolated on the outskirts of your tribe used to mean that you were the most at risk of being attacked by animals or a neighboring tribe, which could lead to early death. We adapted to loneliness to enhance our survival, just like hunger and thirst.*

*Primary relationship insecurity (like problems in a marriage or going through a separation or divorce) can also contribute deeply to uncertainty and a feeling of lack of control over safety.[5] Most people have lost that sense of shared rituals and security in social roles, and that ambiguity can feel unsafe. People with social anxiety have lower heart rate variability, which means they are physically less able to adapt to stress.[6] Sociological factors such as discrimination, racism, and financial uncertainty (especially poverty) also cause significant feelings of unsafety related to the breakdown of social connections.*

*We've also seen that a lifetime of discrimination and being subject to racial profiling is associated with a higher risk of hypertension in Black populations.[7] I suspect it has led to many other long-term health effects besides hypertension, due to the ongoing chronic stress it causes, which underlies (as you've already seen) so many chronic diseases.*

*To send safety signals to your brain, repair familial and social ties, engage in community events, work hard on your personal relationships, and avoid isolating yourself during stress. Physical touch in particular is helpful for sending safety signals to the brain. Even getting an animal companion can trigger safety signals.*

3. **COMPROMISED CONTEXTS.** *Compromised contexts come from the environment you live in, like dangerous urban environments, non-naturalized environments with a lack of green space (separation from nature is inherently stressful), and noise pollution, which potentially keeps people from hearing danger signals, like the approach of a predator.*

   *There is enough evidence to prove that there is a link between environmental noise, sleep disturbances, and cardiovascular disease.[8] Noise pollution increases the amount of signal processing the brain must do in order to differentiate between what is safe and what isn't—constant noise blurs information about possible dangers. It's also just constant arousal in the brain. When we used to live in the woods or on the savanna, it would have been quiet most of the time, unless there were animals nearby. Dark, foggy, smoky, or polluted environments are also dangerous—you can't see what's coming.*

   *Stressful work environments are a part of this category, too. Having tyrannical bosses contributes to generalized uncertainty because you don't know if you're going to keep your job or your resources. Home environments can be super stressful if the people in them are angry or abusive—this can contribute to the entire family's having heightened stress reactivity. Home environments are also stressful if you live in a dangerous neighborhood or your home is not secure.[9]*

   *These environmental stressors can be difficult to remedy because*

## NOISE POLLUTION TRACKING

Peter McBride, a photographer who travels to the quietest places on earth to photograph them, once remarked, "Silence is not the absence of sound, it's the absence of noise."[10] The Grand Canyon at night with no birds or wind has a noise level of about 10 decibels. A quiet room is around 28 to 33 decibels. There is evidence supporting the idea that outside, during the day, humans should not be exposed to a noise level of more than 60 decibels, and at night they should be exposed to no more than 55 decibels of background environmental noise.[11] Normal conversation, a microwave oven, and a laser printer are all about the same, at 55 to 65 decibels. A vacuum cleaner is 62 to 85 decibels. A gas-powered lawn mower is 87 to 92 decibels. A weed trimmer is 94 to 96 decibels, a leaf blower 95 to 105, a chain saw 110, and a snowmobile, firecrackers, and rock concerts are 140 decibels.

You can download decibel meter apps on your phone so you can get a sense of how loud your environment is. Some smartwatches also come with a built-in noise detector and will alert you if environmental noise reaches a damaging level. When you're looking for a new place to live, you can measure the decibels outside to see where they fall, knowing this is going to make a difference in your well-being.

*people usually can't just switch jobs or change their living environments. It may be useful to try to get away from your stressful environment more often, like spending time in nature on the weekends if you live in a big city. Walking through wooded areas can significantly reduce markers of stress hormones in the body and improve markers of immune function.[12] Go on hikes regularly to reconnect with nature, if you are able. Learning coping skills from a counselor or a therapist can also help manage stressful situations you can't change or can't immediately change. Also, if you do have a choice about a place to live or a job to take, you can factor environmental stress into your decision. You can't always know how stressful a situation will be or how dangerous a place will feel, but if you tune into how your body feels in that place, you might get some helpful information.*

Addressing GUTS can significantly lower your foundational stress level, helping to resolve chronic stress and make obvious stressors feel easier and more manageable. It's hard to overstate how much this underlying feeling of unsafety can contribute to chronic stress states; I have seen great success in patients who are able to improve this baseline level of stress.

## Childhood Traumas and Adverse Childhood Events (ACEs)

Childhood traumas can be a profound source of pain that affects adults in complex ways, causing decades of stress that can lead to a multitude of health issues. What you experience as a child shapes your worldview, and it can be difficult to rewind this programming.

It starts at the beginning, even before birth. Your mother's experience of pregnancy was transmitted to you in ways that can affect your temperament and your neurobehavioral development. Infants whose mothers were under high stress while pregnant may show signs of depression, cognitive problems, and irritability. The birth experience can also imprint on you for life. I had a traumatic birth, with a cord prolapse (it wrapped around my neck, strangling me as I was being born). This kind of stress in childbirth can affect your brain development, and I believe it affected mine. Traumatic birth is linked with cognitive issues like attention deficit disorder (ADD). Notably, I'm the only one of my sisters with problems with attention. Some studies show that birth trauma may play a role in the development of ADD in particular,[13] which can then go on to make the rest of life stressful for the neuroatypical person.

Most parents do the best they can to safeguard and protect children, but life itself is traumatic. What happened to you may not seem like a big deal, because often we bury our traumas from childhood to protect ourselves. One way to conceptualize trauma is by thinking of it as divided into two categories—"little-t" and "big-T." Big-T traumas tend to be devastating events that happened to you or your family members, like losing a parent or sibling, or you or one of your family members being abused or harmed. One of my patients had a sibling who died in her sleep from an infection while she was sleeping in the bed next to her, and this contributed to her struggling with PTSD as an adult. That's an example of a big-T trauma.

Little-t traumas are less severe events that nevertheless changed you or shaped your identity. For example, one of my patients had parents who wouldn't let her knock on their bedroom door at night when she was scared as a child, and that created a fear-based identity and has affected her sense of security throughout life. It sounds small, but it created an attachment wound for her.

Someone could have little-t trauma from getting lost for a short time as a child, knowing the family is experiencing problems (marital problems of parents, financial problems, etc.), getting yelled at a lot or criticized, minor bullying at school (major bullying can cause big-T trauma), or really anything else that makes a child feel scared or unsafe for any reason, even if adults don't think it *should* cause those feelings.

Trauma is often a reflection of someone's perception of what happened, as well as how supported they felt after the event. Children feel what they feel and it isn't always reflective of how adults might perceive the situation. Childhood can be an uncertain, frightening, stressful time because children live in a world with no real control over what happens to them.

When I help patients dig deep into their own psychology, we almost always find something, big-T or little-T, that has influenced their life in profound ways. Sometimes it's having a parent with mental illness or a substance abuse issue, and sometimes there's no clear event but instead a constant sense of insecurity or fear because they didn't feel safe as a child. Maybe they felt unlovable or were alone a lot or were told they were stupid or ugly. Even hearing something one time can stick with a child forever.

## Exploring ACEs

ACEs are a particular type of serious big-T trauma that has been studied and can be identified using an ACE questionnaire. ACEs include experiences like sexual abuse, physical abuse, emotional abuse, physical or emotional neglect, witnessing alcoholism or drug use, parental mental illness, parental divorce, or witnessing violence. ACEs are more common than people think. Incredibly, one in four girls and one in thirteen boys was sexually abused as a child, and in 91 percent of those cases, the abuser was someone the child or the child's family knew.[14] That is an ACE that can change the course of a life.

ACEs increase the risk of chronic health problems,[15] including heart disease, obesity, cancer, and autoimmune disease. They increase the likelihood of mental illnesses like depression, PTSD, substance abuse (including alcoholism and opioid misuse), and suicide. They increase the incidence of risky sexual behaviors and STIs, and girls who were sexually abused are two to thirteen times more likely to experience sexual victimization as adults. Anyone who experienced child sexual abuse is twice as likely to experience nonsexual violence in their adult intimate relationships.[16] People with ACEs can also develop behavioral challenges, poor school performance, and underemployment. Early life stress is associated with chronically low heart rate variability that continues into adulthood, and the risk of future disease is dose-dependent: the more trauma, the higher the risk.[17]

It's also important to recognize that there are Protective Childhood Experiences (PCEs), which act as resilience factors that protect individuals from the detrimental effects of ACEs. These include the ability to talk with your family members about your feelings, having the feeling your family supported you during difficult times, enjoying participating in community traditions, feeling like you belonged in high school, feeling supported by your friends, having at least two non-parent adults who genuinely cared about you, and feeling safe and protected by an adult at home.[18] If you suspect you've had adverse childhood experiences, I recommend taking both free online ACE and PCE questionnaires to gain more clarity on your early life experiences. The questions might bring back some difficult memories, but becoming aware of your ACEs can be the first step to resolving the chronic stress they are causing.

The sooner you can identify where you had traumas in your life, the sooner you can begin working on healing those areas. Healing trauma does not happen overnight. It happens over time, and it requires work. Working with a therapist to help you heal can change your life for the better. Traumas operate in the brain like viruses running malware in the background. If you work on reprogramming the brain, you can turn down that background noise and purge, or at least quarantine, the malware so it stops hurting you all the time.

## Discovering Your Core Wound

Whether it's big-T or little-t, your core wound is something you can trace back to childhood that you still carry within your psychology, through adulthood. It might have been a very intense experience, or it might have been something that, on the surface, doesn't appear significant but impacted you intensely—even as an adult, it triggers you and has become a core facet of your personality.

In my case, a series of family traumas that occurred when I was young resulted in a core wound that left me feeling like I had to take care of myself because nobody else would. On some level, I still feel like that, which has resulted in my being independent to a fault. I became a perfectionistic overachiever, and I burned out many times because I didn't know how to ask for help—or, at some level, didn't think help would be available to me.

It's important to understand that we can respond to core wounds in different ways, some of which can appear more adaptive than others. We may engage in addictive or self-harming behaviors, or we may focus on behaviors that, from the outside, seem productive. Sometimes, a core wound might drive both types of behaviors. For example, I believe my core wound inspired my professional ambition. When your coping mechanisms seem to benefit your life, it can be difficult for your ego to let go of them. It's important to recognize this, and to see the difference between strengths you have now and the core wound you haven't healed. You can become attached to your traumas, and it takes work to change how you respond to them. Oftentimes if we do work through them we become even stronger than we were before.

Still, I have seen patients start to make progress and then self-sabotage their healing. One of my patients suffered from a chronic condition and just as she was making enormous shifts and displaying improved energy output, she ignored my advice, pushed herself too hard, and found herself in a surgical suite for an injury she sustained from overexertion. Psychologist and personal growth teacher Dr. Gay Hendricks describes the "upper limit problem"—a phenomenon where, when people start to reach a new level, they bring themselves back down to their comfort zone.[19] Creating change is hard, but sustaining change can be even harder, for psychological reasons.

If your accomplishments are dependent on your internalizing your pain and turning it into success, you may fear that you'll be less successful if you work through your pain. It's useful to recognize that your response to trauma served an important purpose at one point in your life, but it's okay to let go of those behaviors as you grow and heal. The more we transcend our pain and the ego attachment we have to our life experiences, the smarter, more loving, and more joyful our lives become.

You get to keep the strength you have. It was a gift born out of your trauma. But you can still heal the core wound that, despite its gifts, is also still hurting you.

## C-PTSD

You've probably heard of post-traumatic stress disorder, or PTSD. Some people have PTSD from a major, horrible life trauma, but there is another type of PTSD called complex post-traumatic stress disorder, or C-PTSD, that comes from longer-term trauma, like having a parent with borderline personality disorder or addiction throughout your childhood. It's less about one instance than about the environment in which you grew up. I encourage anyone who has suffered from childhood mistreatment, trauma, or neglect to check out the work of Pete Walker, who wrote about complex PTSD.[20]

# Therapy: An Overview

I can't stress enough the value of working with a mental health professional to address trauma and feelings of unsafety. Even if you haven't experienced trauma but you find that you are struggling with a baseline level of stress, seeking help a from a qualified therapist can be life-changing. There are many different approaches to mental health out there, and it's important to find a model and a practitioner that suit your needs. Here are a few types of interventions you might consider:

- **COGNITIVE BEHAVIORAL THERAPY.** Cognitive behavioral therapy (CBT) is based on the idea that psychological problems are, at least in part, based on faulty thought patterns. CBT helps people change their thoughts, recognize distortions in thinking that are creating problems, and learn how to reevaluate their assumptions (cognitive reappraisal).

CBT therapists can also help people recognize their patterns and behaviors, many of which may be automatic, by bringing awareness to them and offering strategies that interrupt those patterns, so people can be more intentional and less reactive. CBT is especially beneficial for people suffering from depression, anxiety, substance abuse, eating disorders, sexual dysfunction, and relationship problems.

- **DIALECTICAL BEHAVIOR THERAPY (DBT).** This is a newer form of therapy that emphasizes mindfulness and learning emotional regulation, becoming tolerant of distressing situations, implementing change-oriented strategies, and developing interpersonal effectiveness. This may be a useful treatment for people who struggle with emotional regulation, addiction, post-traumatic stress disorder, or personality disorders like borderline personality disorder or obsessive-compulsive personality disorder. The primary focus of DBT is emotional regulation.

- **EYE MOVEMENT DESENSITIZATION AND REPROCESSING THERAPY (EMDR).** This is a type of psychotherapy that's traditionally been used for people with PTSD, but it's increasingly being utilized for other issues, from little-t traumas to anxiety. This therapy helps people work through distressing memories while experiencing bilateral eye movements, tapping, or tones to focus the mind on the feelings and sensations that are connected to these memories. There are also EMDR therapists who specialize in complex PTSD.

- **INTERNAL FAMILY SYSTEMS (IFS).** IFS is based on the idea that everyone has different parts inside them that play different roles and perceive situations in different ways. IFS therapy helps people identify their various parts or subpersonalities—such as the manager, the exile, and the firefighter—to help them work through and better understand the reasons for their emotional responses. IFS can be effective for anxiety disorders, depression, and trauma.

- **NEUROFEEDBACK, HYPNOTHERAPY, SOUND HEALING, AND SOMATIC THERAPY** are other types of therapy that may interest you. A patient of mine recommended neurofeedback to me, which improved my cognitive functioning after I suffered from a concussion. Neurofeedback is a great way to use technology to biohack your brain—you are hooked up to sensors and you can see what your brain waves and nervous system electrical signals are doing, so you can learn to feel and manipulate them. I've also found enormous benefit from somatic therapies, which integrate mind and body through movement and touch, as well as hypnotherapy, sound healing, and various kinds of advanced meditation and energy work with skillful healers. There are quite a few holistic modalities out there that require a professional guide. To find what might work for you, do some research on your own and talk to people who have tried various kinds of therapies.

- **OTHER CUTTING-EDGE TRAUMA THERAPIES.** Unresolved trauma can be very energetically draining because the nervous system can remain stuck on hypervigilance and threat mode from an event in the past. Some of the more cutting-edge therapies to explore for treating trauma include Accelerated Experiential-Dynamic Psychotherapy (AEDP), attachment-oriented therapies, Sensorimotor Psychotherapy (SP), Somatic Experiencing (SE), psychedelic-assisted psychotherapy (e.g., ketamine-assisted therapy), and trauma-focused neurofeedback.

Sometimes it can be tough to find a therapist who is the right fit for you. It's so important to work with someone you trust, and someone who sees and respects your identity and experience. You should feel that this person is being truly objective and nonjudgmental, so you can be comfortable revealing the parts of yourself that are hard for you to see. If there's any discomfort in being vulnerable with someone, or if you don't feel safe with them, then they're not the right therapist for you.

## KETAMINE-ASSISTED THERAPY

Ketamine is the first psychedelic to make it into medical practice, and it is proving to be a useful tool for creating more neuroplasticity in the brain. Chronic stress reduces neuroplasticity and makes it harder for people to shift their thoughts and habits. Ketamine can help the brain create new neural connections and new pathways to think about problems more effectively. It's a fascinating drug because it not only reduces depression, anxiety, and pain but also induces an altered state of consciousness characterized by dissociation, or a separation of mind and body. Music is paramount to the experience and can help people to be carried by the journey to parts of their mind that they haven't explored in years.

Ketamine is used in clinics and administered via an IV or through intramuscular injections, or it can be prescribed as sublingual lozenges or an intranasal inhaler that delivers the medicine through mucous membranes in the mouth and nose. I've created a sublingual ketamine protocol that combines lifestyle changes with weekly to biweekly sessions and extensive integration recommendations, including therapy. Before taking any psychedelic medicine, it's important to be in a centered headspace and an environment in which you feel safe and at ease with a qualified practitioner. While the research on ketamine therapy is still evolving, it seems to offer an exciting opportunity for people suffering from depression to heal with greater ease and resolution.

Now that you have a better understanding of the subtle underpinnings of stress and the psychological component of healing, let's take a closer look at how we can transform our physiological experience of stress through biohacking—specifically, how you can counter chronic stress and get more benefit from the stress you experience by incorporating more recovery.

**STRESS RESPONSE BIOHACKS IN THIS CHAPTER**

- Assess whether you have feelings of underlying stress based on a compromised physical body, social network, or environment.

- Track noise pollution in your environment.

- Assess whether you may have childhood trauma or adverse childhood experiences using the ACE questionnaire on my website.

- Try therapy to help you resolve foundational stress, especially CBT, DBT, EMDR, IFS, or any other type of therapy focused on trauma.

# CHAPTER 11

# Biohacking to Recharge

A diamond is just a chunk of coal that did well under pressure.

—Proverb

Many people are so used to the feeling of being stressed that they don't realize the way they feel is not how human bodies are supposed to feel. When I first start working with patients, they often say they aren't under much stress, and it's not until we start going through some assessments that they realize how stressed they really are. Stress may already be impacting their health, not to mention their performance at work, in school, or in sports.

Let's begin by assessing your stress level with a questionnaire. Read through the list of symptoms below and check off everything you have felt or experienced in the last month. There is no scoring system.[1] The purpose of this list is to start bringing your awareness to the ways stress is impacting you right now. If you have a lot of these symptoms, you have a lot of stress. If you don't have many, you're probably doing okay.

*Physical Symptoms*
- o   Headaches
- o   Indigestion

o   Stomachaches
o   Sweaty palms
o   Sleep difficulties
o   Dizziness
o   Back pain
o   Tight neck or shoulders
o   Restlessness
o   Tiredness
o   Ringing in ears

### Behavioral Symptoms

o   Excessive smoking or vaping
o   Bossiness
o   Compulsive gum-chewing
o   Attitude critical of others
o   Grinding teeth at night
o   Overuse of alcohol
o   Compulsive eating
o   Inability to get things done

### Emotional Symptoms

o   Crying
o   Boredom
o   Feeling powerless to change things
o   Easily upset or edgy
o   Ready to explode
o   Overwhelming sense of nervousness, anxiety, or pressure
o   Anger

o   Loneliness

o   Unhappiness for no reason

*Cognitive Symptoms*

o   Trouble thinking clearly

o   Lack of creativity

o   Memory loss

o   Forgetfulness

o   Inability to make decisions

o   Thoughts running away

o   Constant worry

o   Loss of sense of humor

*Spiritual Symptoms*

o   Emptiness

o   Loss of meaning

o   Doubt

o   Problems with forgiveness

o   Martyrdom

o   Magical thinking

o   Loss of direction

o   Cynicism

o   Apathy

o   Needing to prove yourself

o   Lack of intimacy

o   Using people

*Relational Symptoms*

o   Isolation

o   Intolerance

o   Resentment

o   Loneliness

o   Hiding

o   Clamming up

o   Lowered sex drive

o   Nagging

o   Lashing out

o   Fewer contacts with family

o   Distrust

o   Fewer contacts with friends

Another way to assess your stress level is through lab tests, such as morning cortisol, DHEA-S (dehydroepiandrosterone sulfate), and heart rate variability. You may need a functional doctor to order these tests for you. Typically, when you're under a lot of stress, your cortisol can end up too high. High cortisol can make you feel edgy, give you high blood pressure, make your sleep restless, or lead to higher blood sugar levels. If the stress continues without recovery, you may end up with low cortisol or low DHEA. Low cortisol levels can contribute to morning fatigue, low blood sugar, and low blood pressure, all of which make you feel exhausted. DHEA-S helps to produce testosterone and estrogen, so it's important for endocrine health. You may already be tracking your heart rate variability, but if not, try measuring it with wrist-, chest-, or finger-worn devices.

The best assessment of all may be checking in with yourself every morning and tuning in to your body to see how you feel. This can be key to understanding how stress affects you, as well as gauging what you can realistically take on that day. If, after some assessment, you determine that you're under a lot of stress, prioritize recovery. Recovery isn't passive or just about resting. It's the dynamic process of restoring mental and physiological energetic resources.

## Heart Rate Variability to Track Recovery

One great way to assess stress as well as track recovery is through heart rate variability, or HRV. This is a measure of the time between heartbeats, beat-to-beat variation, and how quickly your heart rate returns to normal after it increases. When your heart rate takes a long time to get back to normal after being elevated, that indicates a low HRV and is a sign of chronic stress, low fitness, and low resilience. If your heart rate goes back to normal quickly, that indicates a high HRV and is a sign of good health, high fitness, and physical as well as stress-related resilience.

People have widely varying HRVs. What matters more than the exact number is how the number changes from your baseline, indicating more stress or more recovery. Most important is knowing your normal HRV range and noticing what factors contribute to dropping below it.

There is a lot of tech that can track HRV for you when you sleep and/or when you exercise. For advanced fitness or sleep monitoring wearables (like smartwatches and rings), tracking HRV has become pretty standard. If you want more personalized guidance, I recommend certain closed-loop systems on my website that can monitor heart rate and HRV and prescribe specific interventions (e.g., breathwork practices, breath hold practices, meditation, and mindfulness practices) to improve your numbers for better recovery and resilience. You could also make an appointment with a professional biofeedback therapist, who can use equipment to show you how your heart rate changes as you practice various breathing techniques.

## Improve HRV with Vagus Nerve Stimulation

Heart rate variability is controlled by the vagus nerve, which is a cranial nerve that extends from the brain stem to the abdomen, hugging organs along the way. The vagus nerve communicates information to the heart, lungs, eyes, glands, and gut[2] by carrying signals from these organs to the brain and back. It conveys sensory information about the body's organ systems to the central nervous system, and it influences resting heart rate. Therefore, stimulating the vagus nerve to increase vagal tone (getting that nerve in shape) can increase HRV, improve resilience, and bolster stress recovery. Because your vagus nerve is the moderator of heart rate and HRV, high vagal tone (a fit and adaptable vagus nerve) is a sign of resilience. It all goes together like this:[3]

> High vagal tone = high HRV = low heart rate = good ability to recover, or high resilience
>
> Low vagal tone = low HRV = high heart rate = poor ability to recover, or low resilience

Because of this link between HRV, the vagus nerve, and the parasympathetic nervous system, regular stimulation of the vagus nerve can induce recovery mode by lowering heart rate and ultimately increasing HRV over time. The following strategies for stimulating the vagus nerve might surprise you—they are much easier than exercise and don't sound like stress management, but they work:

- GARGLING. Manipulate your vocal cords to activate the vagus nerve by gargling aggressively with water every morning and evening for about thirty seconds.

- TONGUE SCRAPING. Using a tongue scraper to make yourself gag is a great way to stimulate the vagus nerve.

- **SINGING**. This is an enjoyable vagus nerve stimulator. You don't have to be good at it. Sing in the shower.

- **CHANTING**. Chanting, like saying *om* when you meditate and letting it vibrate through your body, is a good way to stimulate the vagus nerve. A study in the *International Journal of Yoga* found that chanting the word *om* deactivated the stress response.[4]

- **LAUGHING**. Laughing tones your vagus nerve and improves your mood. Watch comedy with friends and family. When one person starts laughing, other people are more likely to get laughing, too. Vagus nerve stimulation for all.

- **CHEWING GUM**. According to research, chewing reduces stress in humans and animals, and gum-chewing reduces unpleasant feelings, helps to reduce the stress response, and stimulates the vagus nerve.[5]

## NEXT-LEVEL VAGUS NERVE STIMULATION: COFFEE ENEMAS

Coffee enemas—or enemas in general—aren't for everyone, but they do stimulate the vagus nerve when the bowel expands, and the caffeine stimulates the gastrointestinal nicotinic acetylcholine receptors, causing an urge to defecate. If you then suppress this urge, you fire up the vagus nerve and build endurance, improving vagal tone over time. I don't recommend doing this without consulting someone who knows how to do it properly—it's beyond the scope of this book to teach you how to do a coffee enema, but suffice it to say that the coffee should be room temperature or cooler. Never use hot coffee!

## Stress Resilience Practices

Practices that optimize mitochondrial function also address recovery by increasing energy for repair and restoration. This impacts HRV. Expert in psychophysiology and HRV (and the cofounder and CSO of Hanu Health) Jay Wiles told me that one of the best ways to achieve lower HRV and improved mitochondrial function is with regular exercise. Training in Zone 2 (light cardio at 70 percent of your maximum heart rate) three times a week for 30 minutes and Zone 5 (Tabata, a type of high intensity HIIT training that pushes you to your maximum heart rate for 20 seconds with 10 seconds of rest) once or twice a week for five to ten minutes can do wonders for lowering your heart rate and raising your HRV. (To calculate the zones first find your maximum heart rate by taking 222 minus your age for Zone 5 and then multiplying that number by 0.7 for Zone 2). Other practices that raise HRV, improve mitochondrial function, and induce recovery include:

- PEMF. This stands for "pulsed electromagnetic field," which can optimize mitochondrial function by directly improving how well mitochondria utilize oxygen. You can buy PEMF mats to lie on or microcurrent devices to use passively. I liken PEMF mats and devices to human body chargers. These devices also help with exercise recovery and injury healing. My favorite brands are on my website.

- SAUNA. Infrared saunas are about 60 degrees Celsius, while wet saunas can get up to 100 degrees Celsius. Both offer benefits for detoxification through sweating and some conditioning benefit through increasing heart rate. They also offer the benefit of vasodilation, which expands blood vessels and improves vagal tone. Heat exposure also activates heat-shock proteins, which can trigger cellular repair.

• **SOCIAL CONNECTION**. Connecting with people we love and trust increases oxytocin in the body, which creates a felt sense of safety. Oxytocin, a hormone released in response to physical touch and feelings of love, is a natural antioxidant and anti-inflammatory, so connection and touch (massage, cuddling, sex) can improve physical as well as mental recovery.

## Breathing Exercises

Because the breath directly affects heart rate and HRV, breathing exercises are some of the fastest ways to intervene in the stress response. From traditional pranayama practices of yoga to modern techniques like the 4–7–8 breath developed by Dr. Andrew Weil, breathing exercises are an easy and accessible stress hack.

Belly breathing, also called diaphragmatic breathing, is one of my favorite techniques. Belly breathing uses the diaphragm, a dome-shaped muscle below your lungs. Belly breathing increases vagal tone and can trigger the parasympathetic response, turning off stress signals and inducing calm. It helps your lungs empty more completely, loosens tight muscles, and decreases blood pressure. Rapid shallow chest breathing, by contrast, can trigger the sympathetic nervous system and impair emotional regulation by increasing cortisol release, heart rate, and sweating. To your body, rapid breathing feels like fear.

Here's how to do belly breathing: Lie down in a comfortable position. Put one hand on your belly just below your ribs, the other hand on your chest. Take a deep breath through your nose but let your belly expand under your hand, rather than your chest. Try to keep your chest still. To exhale, push the air out with your abdominal muscles. If you breathe in and out with pursed lips, as if you're whistling, you can really feel your belly moving more (this is called pursed-lip breathing). Do this three to ten times to feel calmer and more relaxed.[6]

Some other effective breathing techniques:

- RESONANT FREQUENCY BREATHING. There are apps and wearables that can help you find your resonant frequency breathing rate, but a simplified way to do this is to breathe in for 4 counts and breath out for 6 counts. Start with three to five minutes a day and gradually work your way up to ten to fifteen minutes a day.

- ALTERNATE-NOSTRIL BREATHING. This is a traditional yoga practice that's effective for recovering from stress. Sit quietly and take a few breaths to relax, then put your right thumb on your right nostril and close it. Close your eyes and exhale fully and slowly through your left nostril. Once you have exhaled completely, release your right nostril, and put your ring finger on the left side of your nose and close your left nostril. Breathe in deeply and slowly from the right side. Try to keep your breaths smooth and continuous. Once you have inhaled completely, exhale through your right nostril. Release your ring finger and close your right nostril with your thumb again. Breathe in fully, then exhale fully from your left nostril. Repeat this process for at least ten minutes for the best effect.

- 4–7–8 BREATHING. This pattern of breathing puts you right into parasympathetic nervous system mode—it can stop an anxiety or panic attack. Inhale for a count of four, hold your breath for a count of seven, then exhale slowly for a count of eight. Repeat as needed.

- BOX BREATHING. This is an easy exercise you can do discreetly, anywhere, when you need to calm down. Inhale for a count of four, hold for a count of four, exhale for a count of four, hold for a count for four. Repeat as needed.

# Biohacking Sleep and Circadian Rhythm

Sleep is probably the most important recovery strategy at your disposal. Circadian rhythm is your internal clock that cues you to go to sleep, wake up, eat, fast, move, or rest, according to internal and external natural rhythm cues (like sunrise and sunset). A healthy circadian rhythm translates to good sleep, and good sleep promotes healing, consolidates memories, and cleanses the brain. The brain has its own waste removal system, called the glymphatic system, and it kicks in and cleans house during deep sleep.[7]

Back sleepers may have lower sleep quality, with more light sleep and less REM and deep sleep, than side sleepers. Neck angle is also important. Spending more than two hours per night on your back or with your neck in a non-horizontal position (sleeping in any position where your head is not in line with your spine) decreases glymphatic system function,[8] so pay attention to your sleep position and head support.

Here are a few ways to normalize circadian rhythm and maximize quality sleep for optimal stress recovery:

- **REGULATE YOUR SLEEP AND WAKE CYCLES** approximately with the cycles of light and dark or sunset and sunrise. Deep sleep is the most restorative, and you get the majority of it in the first half of the night. Get to bed by ten P.M. and avoid the cortisol surge that can happen around eleven P.M. that can keep you awake for another few hours.

- **GET FULL-SPECTRUM SUNLIGHT IN THE MORNING** and watch the sunset at night when you can, to regulate your circadian rhythms and associated hormones. Your body will respond to these natural light cues.

- **LIMIT EXPOSURE TO BLUE LIGHT AT NIGHT** by reducing screen time. Blue light mimics sunlight, so it tricks your body into thinking it should stay awake. This suppresses melatonin and activates the suprachiasmatic nucleus in the brain, sending wakefulness signals that affect circadian timing and sleep physiology, causing hyper-arousal at night. Poor sleep affects alertness, so the more blue light we get at night, the less alert we are during the day. Some smartphones have "night mode" settings to block their own blue light at night, or you can use blue-light-filtering apps. You can also block blue light physically, with blue-blocking glasses you can wear at night around the house, or buy blue-blocking screen shields to use after sundown.

- **KEEP A CONSISTENT SLEEP SCHEDULE**. Maintaining sleeping and waking times within about a ninety-minute window helps regulate your circadian rhythm.

- **CREATE A CONSISTENT BEDTIME ROUTINE**. Do the same things at the same times in the same order each night, like taking a shower, washing your face, brushing your teeth, reading, meditating, and turning out the lights.

- **MAKE YOUR ROOM COMFORTABLE AND RELAXING**. Sleep in a clean room with good air quality and comfortable bedding.

- **BLOCK OUT ALL LIGHT AND SOUND** with blackout curtains or a sleep mask and earplugs.

- **USE ESSENTIAL OILS** like chamomile and lavender before sleep. Rub them between your palms and cup your palms over your face, or put some in a diffuser in your room.

- **USE SUPPLEMENTS THAT ENCOURAGE GOOD SLEEP**, like melatonin, magnesium, glycine, valerian, passionflower, or GABA.

**SLEEP HACKING AND TRACKING**

There are a lot of devices and apps that track sleep and provide information about your sleep length and quality, and many of my patients have experienced significant benefits from using these. Sleep-tracking devices show you how long you actually slept, not just how long you were in bed. Some can track how much time you spent in different sleep stages, so you can determine whether you got enough restorative deep sleep. You can also find white-noise apps to improve sleep. Certain binaural beats (1 to 4 Hz in the delta range) are popular for helping people fall asleep, get better sleep quality, and spend more time in deeper sleep. Other sleep-supportive devices include acupressure mats and infrared heating mats for relaxing after a strenuous day. Some can even use sound to diagnose sleep apnea (but I recommend all clients who snore or have significant sleep problems get a clinical sleep study).

- **DON'T DRINK ALCOHOL OR CAFFEINE** in the evening. If you have any trouble sleeping, try to cut off caffeine consumption before two P.M., or even better, before noon.

- **TRACK YOUR SLEEP** using wrist or ring wearables. There are even mattresses and mattress toppers that track sleep.

## Recovery Through Mindfulness

Practicing mindfulness can retrain your brain to manage stress better. As defined by renowned mindfulness researcher Jon Kabat-Zinn, mindfulness is the process of "paying attention, on purpose, in the present moment, and nonjudgmentally, to the unfolding of experience, moment by moment."[9] Mindfulness interventions focus on cultivating awareness, not striving to change something but accepting the experience of the present moment. Mindfulness practices improve vagal tone and signal the body to enter parasympathetic mode. It's mental fitness training, as you learn to become more aware of how you feel and can observe your thoughts and sensations.

Research shows that mindfulness-based stress reduction has a host of health benefits, including improving the body's natural immune response and reducing C-reactive protein, a marker of inflammation.[10] Mindfulness treatments can be just as effective as psychological and psychiatric interventions, especially for depression and pain conditions, and they may also be useful for people trying to quit smoking or overcome other addictions.[11]

It doesn't take any training to practice mindfulness. Simply set an intention every morning to be mindful during the day. An intention is like an arrow you shoot toward where you want your day to go. Throughout the day, work on being in the present moment when you feel your mind slipping into the past or future.

You can also choose to be mindful during certain activities, like brushing your teeth. Notice the entire process—turning on the water, pushing out the toothpaste onto the toothbrush, how it feels to brush every part of your mouth. You could do this while walking your dog, exercising, even eating lunch. Slow down, sit down, pause, breathe, and really taste your food. Other opportunities to practice mindfulness: doing laundry, waiting in line, sitting in traffic, or anything else that feels rote or boring. Try to move away from the idea of boredom and toward the notion of presence. You don't need to do it all the time. Just occasionally, pause and be present for your life. That's mindfulness. It's not complex.

Every time I go outside, no matter what I'm doing, no matter where I'm going, I take a moment to look around, notice the trees, the colors, the wind, the way the sun feels on my skin. I've become so much more present for my life because of these practices. Mindfulness makes you more aware of your thoughts, your feelings, your emotions, your reactions, your triggers. You can learn to create a space where you have a say in how you react to things, and that is a superpower. You don't have to be reactive. You don't have to be entertained every second of your life. You don't have to constantly reach for something to make you feel better. Honestly, that is what makes so many people unhappy. If you can just be where you are, no matter how you feel, then you will become more resilient to all sorts of feelings, thoughts, and experiences, including the negative ones, and they won't have so much power over you.

## Meditation: The Ultimate Recovery Tool

If you really want to become adept at stress recovery, learn how to meditate and do it daily. Meditation is a technique, or a range of different techniques, that trains your mind to regulate your attention, perception, and emotions, and helps to bring your body back into a state of homeostasis by regulating your heart rate, breathing rate, blood pressure, and other basic bodily functions.[12] Meditation can help you to find an inner sense of peace, balance, clarity, and sensory awareness that is extremely beneficial for recovery. The goal of meditation is to achieve a state of equanimity that isn't "good" or "bad" but is simply a nonreactive state of being in the present moment. Everyone benefits from meditation differently, but I find that a regular meditation practice helps me improve my attention and allows me to focus more easily on my work. It's been my best weapon against stress.

There are many types of meditation. I personally like loving-kindness meditation, which focuses on developing compassion for yourself and others. This is one of the first types of meditation that ever really stuck with me. It's great for beginners because it's simple. Guided loving-kindness meditations are easy to find on meditation apps.

Try whatever technique sounds appealing. Just sit, or be mindful, or go outside and connect with sunrise and sunset, preferably barefoot, and ground yourself. You can do a ten-to-fifteen-minute morning or evening practice, or you can be mindful as you do yoga poses or breathing exercises.

Consistency in your recovery practice is more important than the technique you use. Put yourself on a schedule. Once a week, you could do a longer session, or go on a hike, or do a twenty-hour fast, or just honor one day a week (like a Sabbath or Shabbat) as a holy day that you spend being quiet and mindful. You might designate a digital detox day where you don't use any technology. Every two weeks I write down either full moon intentions, which are things I want to bring into my life, or new moon intentions, which are things I want to let go of in my life. Writing my intentions is a kind of mindfulness practice for me. Monthly, you might take your practice deeper, like trying a three-day digital detox in nature or attempting a twenty-four-hour fast. Quarterly, you could aim to connect your practice with your community by attending a sound healing session or some kind of group ritual around the solstices and equinoxes.

I believe it's important for people to get into their communities as much as possible, because this anchors them to where they are in the world. This is surprisingly restorative. Solstices and equinoxes are nice to celebrate in groups because they aren't attached to any religion, but if you are involved with a religious group, religious holidays also offer a wonderful way to integrate spirit and community. Whatever the occasion, these are powerful opportunities to release stress and find meaning and purpose in your life.

## Other Stress Recovery Interventions

There are so many ways to initiate recovery mode. Here are some of the recovery interventions I have found to be effective for my patients and students as well as for myself:

- **ACUPUNCTURE AND ACUPOINT STIMULATION.** One recent study showed that acupuncture can decrease the stress response and induce a short-term rise in HRV.[13] I like acupressure mats, which are cheap and effective ways to stimulate acupressure points on your back. It's one of my best hacks for relieving stress, although acupuncture sessions with a trained acupuncturist are the most potent acupuncture-based stress reducers.

- **EFT.** Emotional freedom technique, more commonly called tapping, is a practice that involves tapping with your fingers in a particular pattern of acupressure points on your face, on your neck, and under your arm. It seems simple, but multiple studies have shown that tapping reduces markers of stress, including the release of cortisol.[14] How does it work? Scientists aren't completely sure. From an Eastern perspective, it may manipulate energy along meridians, similar to acupuncture. Others posit that it might release pain-relieving and calming chemicals, or that it redirects attention from stressful thoughts. There are many instructional tapping videos on You-Tube.

- **TOUCH.** Human touch activates touch receptors under the skin that can decrease blood pressure, heart rate, and cortisol levels. It also releases endocannabinoids and oxytocin, both of which are endogenous opioids (opioids the body makes internally) that promote relaxation. You can get this benefit from hugs and cuddling with loved ones or getting massage or bodywork from a professional.

- **CBD.** CBD, or cannabidiol, seems to have a positive therapeutic effect, relieving anxiety, depression, and stress; reducing pain; improving sleep; and even helping people recover from addictions through its action on the body's endocannabinoid system. It's controversial, mostly because it is (1) made from cannabis, even though it doesn't contain THC, the substance that makes you "high," and (2) it's trendy and people are hyping it up and selling it with claims it can do everything. The research on CBD is ongoing, but the data we do have suggests it increases neurogenesis in the brain and relieves stress symptoms, at least in mice. Quality is important here, so be selective when sourcing.

Recovering from chronic stress may feel like an intimidating project, but it's one that will pay dividends in an improved quality of life now and increased healthspan later.

## Cultivating the Qualities of Resilient Personalities

Recovering from stress is about hacking your physiology, but it's also about shifting your perspective. Some people are easily impacted by stress and others aren't. What makes some people naturally more resilient to stress? Researchers have identified specific qualities and traits that anyone can cultivate for better stress resilience.

While you may or may not have some of these traits naturally, you can cultivate them through practice. These qualities include:

- **COURAGE**. The ability to confront and overcome fear or uncertainty and find strength in the face of pain or grief.

- **CONSCIENTIOUSNESS**. Being careful, diligent, efficient, and organized and taking your obligations seriously.

- **LONG-TERM GOAL SETTING**. Visualizing your future and taking action to move toward your goals.

- **OPTIMISM**. Staying positive and believing that no matter what happens, you will be okay.

- **CREATIVITY**. Approaching problems in unconventional ways to find solutions.

- **CONFIDENCE**. Believing you have the ability to overcome adversity.

- **EXCELLENCE**. Striving to be the best you can be in all your endeavors.

When you build these qualities within yourself, you create a life for yourself that is full of challenges and adversity, but also joy and rewards. Other ways to build resilience include:

- **FOSTERING HEALTHY RELATIONSHIPS** and making connections with supportive people. This could be family, a social group, a church group or other spiritual group, or any group of like-minded, inspiring people. Find your tribe.

- **WORKING TOWARD YOUR GOALS**. Whether you want to learn the piano, get a PhD, or lose twenty pounds, working toward your goals teaches you resilience because progress is not linear and you will always have to contend with obstacles and difficulties. When you achieve goals, you increase your confidence and sense of control over your life. And, even if you fail, if you have a growth mindset in which you can see any circumstance as an opportunity to learn and improve.

- **TAKING CARE OF YOURSELF**. When you commit to cultivating a loving and supportive relationship with yourself, you will get to know yourself better and you will gain confidence in your own strengths, talents, and abilities. Confidence in your own abilities is necessary for resilience. Someone once told me when I was feeling defeated, "If you don't believe in yourself, no one will." This stuck with me and helped me overcome my fears.

- **HAVING A SENSE OF PURPOSE.** What do you live for? If you feel that you have a purpose, you are likely to be healthier, happier, and more resilient in the face of stress; have a higher quality of life; and enjoy more years living it.[15] A 2019 study published in the *Journal of the American Medical Association* found that, of 6,985 adults in the U.S. over fifty years old, those who felt like they had a purpose in their lives were the longest lived and were less likely to die from heart, circulatory, or digestive diseases. Those who ranked purpose low on their list of priorities were 2.43 times more likely to die by the end of the study.[16] To help you find yours, check out the Dharma Inquiry on my website, inspired by my friend Daniel Schmachtenberger, a social philosopher, podcaster, and entrepreneur.[17]

- **TAKING RESPONSIBILITY.** People who take full responsibility for their own lives tend to be much more resilient and happier. In psychology, having an "internal locus of control" means you believe you have control over what happens to you. Research shows that people with an internal locus of control tend to be happier with their lives, have better mental health, and be more resilient in the face of adversity.[18]

- **ENGAGING WITH LIFE.** Look for ways to grow. Be curious, explore, travel. Meet new people. Try new things. Learn consistently. Engaging with life will bring you joy and sorrow. It's not easy, but easy doesn't build resilience.

- **HAVING GRATITUDE.** Learn to truly appreciate who you are, what you have, and who is on this journey with you. Keeping a gratitude journal can be incredible for mental health.

# The Hero's Journey

The hero's journey is a concept in mythology first recognized and called out by author Joseph Campbell in his many books on the subject. Essentially, a hero is called to adventure and goes through a series of stages. At first, the hero refuses the call, then meets with a mentor, crosses a threshold, faces tests, makes friends, fights enemies, approaches a literal or metaphorical cave where they must face their shadow self, reaches a climax on their journey, gets something good, refuses the chance to return home, then ultimately goes back home, changed by the journey and now existing on a higher plane. Typically, the hero is described as a "he," but obviously, women go through this same hero's journey, and it almost sounds demeaning to call it a "heroine's journey." We are heroes, too.

The hero's journey is a metaphor for how each one of us engages with life and eventually finds meaning through facing hardship, learning from it, growing wiser, and ultimately understanding why we are here. The journey is naturally filled with stressors, but the hero perseveres and eventually prevails.

You may already have felt you are on this journey as you've been reading this book, but if you haven't thought about it that way yet, why not start now? Gaining clarity on your goals and then setting out to achieve them is a way to begin the adventure. I've included below some of the questions you can ask yourself to figure out where you are headed in your life. Consider each one of these seriously. You might want to write down your answers so you can organize your thoughts. These are open-ended but serious questions that can help you discover, explore, pursue, and commit to a purpose in life. Ask yourself:

- What do you want?

- When do you want it?

- Why do you want it?

- Who would you be if you accomplished this?

- What will it cost you to get it?

- What will it cost you if you don't get it?

- How will you feel if you achieve it? (Visualize this.)

- How will you feel if you don't achieve it? (Visualize this.)

- What are your *true goals*? Not goals imposed on you by society or the expectations of others according to who they think you are, or because of your gender or profession.

- If you let go of what everyone else thinks, what would you really want to do?

Once you know what your true desires really are, you can set out with a purpose. Your goal can be big or little, but it should feel like *you*. This is your journey, your adventure, your resilience training. Use all the tools you have, stay focused, give yourself time to recover, then get back at it. Your resilience will grow exponentially, and your quality of life will soar. Be the main character in your unique story.

- Assess your stress.

*Strategies to improve vagal tone to increase HRV*

- Vocal cord vibration
- Chanting
- Laughing
- Chewing gum

*Recovery strategies*

- Exposure to pulsed electromagnetic fields
- Sauna
- Address trauma
- Connect physically with loved ones
- Practice kindness and compassion
- Track your HRV to determine how well you are recovering from stress
- Try a new breathing technique, like alternate-nostril breathing, 4–7–8 breathing, or box breathing
- Hack your circadian rhythm
- Watch the sunrise and sunset
- Don't expose yourself to blue light after sundown
- Institute a consistent sleep schedule and bedtime routine
- Clean your bedroom
- Sleep with blackout curtains
- Use essential oils for sleep, especially chamomile and lavender
- Try melatonin, magnesium, glycine, and/or GABA before bed
- Track your sleep
- Work on mindfulness
- Try any type of meditation
- Get an acupuncture treatment or try an acupoint stimulation mat

- Try EFT (tapping)

- Take a CBD supplement

- For a more intensive stress intervention, check out my HPA axis dysfunction protocol on my website

- Assess whether you have the qualities of a resilient personality

- Work on improving your resilience by building your supportive social connections, working toward goals, taking care of yourself, having a sense of purpose, taking responsibility for your actions and life, engaging with life, and having gratitude for what you have now

- Think about your own hero's journey and what your life's purpose is

- If you feel you need a more aggressive and comprehensive recovery strategy, please see the **HPA Axis Protocol** on my website. This protocol lays out a detailed prescription for chronic stress and burnout, so you can recover and get back to baseline. It can take some time, and that's okay. It's worth the effort to reclaim your resilience.

## PART V

# PLUGGING IN YOUR BATTERIES

# CHAPTER 12

# The Hormone-Energy Connection

Women are biologically primed for connection—whether that be through caring for family members, building companies, or creating change in their communities. Counter to the patriarchal belief that our hormones are a liability, our biology gives us superpowers. Women are born with the generative power to create and nurture life, and hormones play an important role in this biological imperative. Whether or not you have children, fertility is a biomarker of health, and our mitochondria are central to this function because they play a central role in making sex hormones, including estrogen and progesterone.

Our hormones are a window into our cellular programming. Understanding how our hormones affect our bodies opens the door for biohacking our way to better health. With excess stress, our mitochondria will redirect our resources to survival and our hormonal cycle can be disrupted. When stress resolves, our mitochondria reestablish our cycle. All of these messages are sent through hormonal signaling. This is the crux of why understanding your hormones is so important for your long-term health and reproductive capacity. Hormones are the connection between the energy we make and how we live our lives each day.

## Making Sense of Your Menstrual Cycle

A woman's rhythms are cyclical—this is one of the primary ways our hormones differ from those of men—and there is no more obvious sign of our cycle than menstruation. And yet, somehow, something so foundational to women's health is often regarded as embarrassment. For women, a "normal" life involves bleeding from the vagina about a quarter of each month during our fertile years, and we have both normalized and suppressed the fact that women bleed quietly, privately—and often endure quite a bit of pain—every month, for decades of our lives. During this time, we are still expected to work, care for our families, and do everything else we normally do. To talk about it openly would be to subject ourselves to ridicule, or worse.

As young girls, often not even teenagers yet, we suddenly have to adjust to this new ritual of bleeding and the cramps, bloating, and mood swings that often accompany it, all the while attending school and pretending like nothing has changed. Pretending we're not terrified of an "accident" that might mean someone will *know we are bleeding*. Then, one day, when that bleeding stops for good, we have to adjust all over again to a different hormonal milieu, physiological changes, and another type of stigma.

Women have always had to biohack their cycles. We essentially invented tampons (a man invented the modern version but women were hacking the concept for centuries before that). We invented pads—an eighteen-year-old Black woman named Mary Beatrice Davidson Kenner first came up with the idea of a belt that held a sanitary napkin in place, in 1957, although as you can probably imagine, she had a hard time getting anybody to produce it. We've had to try to calculate when we're ovulating through all kinds of low-tech hacks like tracking body temperature and examining cervical mucus, whether that's because we're trying to get pregnant or because we're trying not to. We've had to listen carefully to our bodies, receiving their data, and devise hacks that allow us to stay in control of them.

Today, we have the benefit of technology. Period-tracking apps can help you know where you are in your cycle, so that you can adjust your workflow, social life, stress management, exercise, and diet to optimize the benefits of each phase. No more surprises. You can buy luteinizing hormone (LH) strips on Amazon in packs of fifty that test your urine to reveal whether you're having an LH spike. If there's a spike, you're probably ovulating and fertile. There are wearables that monitor your temperature and can help predict your ovulation window as well.

But low-tech hacks (like monitoring your cervical mucus to see how it changes when you ovulate) can still be useful, especially when we sync up with the cycles of nature. In fact, paying attention to your body's cycle can also help you feel more in tune with the cycles of the natural world. When we notice this, we can grow in self-awareness and deepen our respect for and connection with our own biology.

I like to think of the cycles of menstruation in terms of the cycles of the seasons. Menstruation is like the body's winter. Fertility pauses as the uterine lining sheds and the body rests. The follicular phase is similar to the body's spring. The uterine lining begins to build and create fertile ground. The follicles ripen, much like seeds germinating. Summer is our ovulation, when the plants are ripe and fruiting and we are most fertile. The luteal phase is akin to fall, when the leaves change color and drop. If you don't get pregnant, the body begins winding down and preparing to rest.

In the Ojibwe and Yurok Indigenous tribes, menstruation is called "moon time,"[1] and it's considered to be a powerful phase for a woman to focus on herself, let go of negative emotions, rest, and reflect. Interestingly, when I started tracking my emotional state and my period, I found a correlation between carrying negative emotions and heavy periods. Your period can be a window into your life when you realize that hormones play a role in negative emotions and stress plays a role in hormone imbalances. When the body is stressed, the mitochondria make the decision to direct energy resources to survival over reproduction, and this can contribute to sex hormone imbalances and irregular periods. Remember, the body doesn't prioritize fertility if it feels it's under threat.

While I like thinking about the menstrual cycle as mimicking the seasons, of course it's also more complex than that. Let's take a closer look at the phases of a standard menstrual cycle to get a better sense of what's going on inside your body throughout the month and how your cycle can influence your work, social life, stress, fitness, and metabolism.

### MENSTRUATION: STARTS ON DAY ONE

Your period starts on day one of your cycle and typically lasts until about day six. During the start of your period, your estrogen and

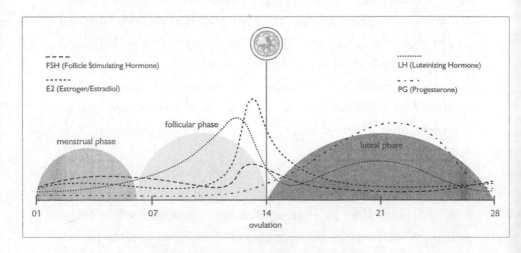

*Figure 1: Phases of the menstrual cycle*

Source: https://helloclue.com/articles/cycle-a-z/the-menstrual-cycle-more-than
-just-the-period

progesterone are at their lowest and the lining of the uterus sheds. In your work and in your social life, this is a great time for reflection, evaluation, and integration of everything that has happened to you in the past month. Your physical energy may be lower during the first half of your period, so don't be surprised if you aren't feeling particularly ambitious or social and a warm bath sounds more inviting than going out with friends. This is a time of rest and recovery and a fertile pause as the body restores, knowing it may need more active creation energy later. Rest without guilt, knowing that high-energy, outward-facing performance time is coming.

When it comes to your fitness, because your hormones are low (and more closely resemble a man's hormonal makeup), it isn't necessarily a bad time for physical performance. Higher hormone levels in the luteal phase can sometimes be more problematic for athletic performance, which is why you feel the most tired on the first day of your period, but a few days in, you will have more energy. Women have run marathons while menstruating, so don't worry if you have a race or a big ride scheduled. You may perform better in sports, but listen to your body. If it says you need rest, then rest.

Because estrogen is the lowest during the menstrual phase, it's best to eat lower-carb during this time. By the end of menstruation, as you are heading into the follicular phase, you may be game for some light intermittent fasting, but only if you're not feeling too stressed.

You may feel more stressed during this time because your levels of the stress hormone cortisol are elevated. High cortisol can make you more insulin resistant, which can make it harder to burn fat and make you more likely to experience blood sugar spikes if you eat high-carb. Gentle exercise is one of the best antidotes to stress. Pay attention and track your flow so you can see what makes it heavier or lighter—this is actionable information. I've noticed that I have heavier periods when I have experienced a lot of stress or have not exercised very much during the preceding month.

Iron-rich foods are also important now. Aim for foods like grass-fed beef, fish, leafy greens, liver, and dark chocolate, and combine them with vitamin C–rich foods (bell peppers, citrus fruits, strawberries, broccoli) to aid in absorption. Taking vitamin D can also help you absorb more iron. Extra antioxidants (berries, red cabbage, citrus) and anti-inflammatory foods (extra-virgin olive oil, turmeric, ginger) can help to relieve some period pain. If you are eating iron-rich foods or taking iron supplements and you have persistently low iron or ferritin levels (ideally, ferritin should be greater than 75 ng/dL), this could be due to a copper deficiency. Copper is required to absorb iron in the gut, so if levels are low it can be tough to get enough iron.

## THE FOLLICULAR STAGE: DAYS SEVEN TO THIRTEEN

During this time, your body starts making more estrogen and progesterone. At work and socially, you'll begin to feel more active, assertive, outward facing, and achievement oriented. This is the time to generate new ideas, brainstorm, initiate projects, and exercise your creativity; it is your planning-organizing-execution stage. You might also find you have a greater stress tolerance and a higher pain threshold, and your immunity is strongest in this phase.

Fitness-wise, since your progesterone is still relatively low, you can put on muscle more easily, so make gains with strength training. You can push harder since you will have extra glycogen to burn, and you can challenge yourself with higher intensities, heavier weights, and fewer reps (like one to six reps of heavier weights when you would normally do seven to twelve reps with lower weights). In addition, you'll have faster reaction time, so this is the phase in which to do HIIT classes, do hill sprints, beat your personal record on runs or rides, and increase your one-rep max while lifting heavy weights.

As estrogen starts to rise during the follicular phase, you become more sensitive to insulin, which means that you can more easily access carbs and burn them. Increasing your carb intake will help you push for better performance in the gym.

If you don't exercise or if you are overweight, a little intermittent fasting (e.g., fourteen to sixteen hours) can be a good option now, because it acts a lot like exercise in your body in the way it cleans out the damaged cellular parts (autophagy). Fasting creates a kind of beneficial stress in the body that builds metabolic resilience, as long as you aren't piling it on top of other stressors.

Don't fast if you are a heavy exerciser. Women who exercise and fast risk underfueling, which can cause multiple hormonal systems to become imbalanced, increasing cortisol and interfering with the healthy production of estrogen, thyroid hormones, and kisspeptin (a hormone instrumental in puberty and fertility).

## OVULATION: AROUND DAYS THIRTEEN TO FIFTEEN

Estrogen peaks before ovulation. Luteinizing hormone (LH) and follicle-stimulating hormone (FSH) also spike around this time, causing the ovaries to release an egg sometime between days thirteen and fifteen. Estrogen begins to decline following ovulation, making the body a little less insulin sensitive (which means you won't tolerate carbs as well).

In your work and social life, this is the moment when you may find you feel the most creative, energized, articulate, magnetic, and receptive. This is prime time for dating, promoting work projects, making pitches, doing sales calls, and making presentations. You will have an increased ability to connect, collaborate, and communicate. Just be careful not to overload yourself with work or other stressors, as your immunity is a bit lower now.

Higher estrogen levels prior to ovulation means there is a greater risk for tendon injuries in sports, so be more careful in your workouts. Progesterone starts going up after ovulation, decreasing anabolic capacity, which means you may or may not feel like hitting it as hard in the gym as you did during your follicular phase. How hard you exercise depends on how you feel, but instead of pushing yourself to extremes, focus on moderate effort.

Your body is the most insulin sensitive when estrogen is highest, which means your body prefers carbs for fuel during the days before you ovulate. Make sure to include lots of fiber and phytonutrient-rich, slow-metabolizing carbs like green veggies, cruciferous vegetables, root vegetables, and berries, because these will help you metabolize excess estrogen. Pumpkinseed and flax are also helpful here with estrogen metabolism. Your increased energy needs during this phase will also slightly elevate your calorie burn by 100 to 150 calories.

## EARLY LUTEAL STAGE: DAYS FIFTEEN TO TWENTY-THREE

If you didn't get pregnant during ovulation, your body begins to produce more progesterone. Although estrogen drops after ovulation, it starts to steadily rise again, but this time progesterone rises alongside it. This is why the luteal phase is called the high-hormone phase. Progesterone and estrogen have opposite effects on insulin sensitivity (because estrogen promotes insulin sensitivity, but progesterone counteracts estrogen, reducing insulin sensitivity), so it's hard to predict how your metabolism will behave. In general, you want to eat lower-carb because your body uses more fat for fuel during this phase.

This is a time to be more receptive to your body's needs. You may need to rest or take a gentler approach to work. You can also begin to turn inward as progesterone rises. It's a good time for planning and reflecting. Although progesterone is high, so is estrogen, and that can potentially cause inflammation (though everyone's fluctuations are a bit different). This is where PMS symptoms first come into play.

You may find you need to ease up on the cardio, fasting, and metabolic challenges like eating a ketogenic diet. Emphasize low to moderate intensity strength and endurance exercise. Try long hikes at a moderate pace. For weight lifting, focus on lifting light or moderate loads with higher reps (seven to fifteen). Your body prefers burning fat in this stage, so lower carb eating will be the best for fueling your less intense training schedule.

Your easy access to carbs is declining now, so you won't be able to access the energy for higher-intensity sports without extra glucose. In the absence of glucose with heavy exercise, the body could start to catabolize muscle, which can cause muscle wasting over time. A way to counter this now is to take two to three grams of essential amino acids (EAAs)—a group of three amino acids your body uses to make muscle—before and after exercise. I find tablets you can swallow whole far more palatable than the powdered-drink forms of BCAAs, which invariably taste bad.

Your progesterone-fueled higher core temperature and increased catabolism (muscle loss) mean you'll get tired sooner, especially when it's hot. You will likely sweat more and can lose too much salt. A lot of women feel bloated in this phase but actually need more salt, not less. This is when electrolytes are your friend. You may not feel as thirsty in this phase, so it's important to maintain hydration (aim for about 64 ounces of water a day) rather than relying on thirst to alert you.

In general, the luteal phase is when we feel less energized, feel hungrier, have more food cravings, and have a desire to eat more. To counteract the hunger and cravings, make sure to get enough protein, fat, and fiber at every meal. Don't beat yourself up because you're having cravings. Just do your best to not use your period as an excuse to binge on junk food, because you're not as insulin sensitive and you're more likely to get bloated and experience bigger peaks and dips in blood sugar.

## LATE LUTEAL STAGE: DAYS TWENTY-FOUR TO TWENTY-EIGHT

Estrogen and progesterone start to decline leading up to menstruation, and cortisol levels increase during the late luteal phase. This means you may feel hungrier, moodier, and more stressed out. At least 50 percent of women experience symptoms of PMS in this phase.

This is a time to hunker down to complete projects and focus on tying up loose ends. Shift your attention to detail-oriented work that doesn't require you to be "on" around people. While exercise is one of the best antidotes to stress, you may feel like reducing the intensity and volume of exercise. This is a time for yoga, gentle Pilates, mobility work, and prioritizing recovery. For cardio, long walks or easy jogs are all you need.

Less estrogen means less serotonin in the brain, making you more likely to feel anxious or depressed. To counteract this, choose foods higher in tryptophan (turkey, tahini, bananas, spirulina, sesame seeds) to provide you with the building blocks for making serotonin, which will improve your mood and help you sleep better. A sweet, healthy whole-food treat can also make you feel better by boosting serotonin. Sesame and sunflower seeds can help boost progesterone. My favorite treat is a tahini-stuffed date with a little dark chocolate melted on top, sprinkled with salt.

## The Stages of Your Hormonal Life

Each month is a cycle, but so is your whole life. Every decade or two in a woman's life, hormones shift dramatically, and hormonal fluctuations change you. And just as with your menstrual cycle, there are many ways you can intervene to track and hack these life stages.

### PUBERTY: USING YOUTH TO YOUR ADVANTAGE

Puberty is the first major transition young girls will go through, and sometimes it can feel like the whole world is crashing down around them. Girls going through puberty need more calories because they are

## HACK YOUR PMS WITH SUPPLEMENTS

PMS symptoms are usually most pronounced during the five days leading up to your period, but supplements can help mitigate the symptoms. These are the supplements I've found to be most helpful, personally and for my patients:

- **CALCIUM** (500 mg once or twice a day) is one of the most important supplements for women with PMS or PMDD. Calcium helps to regulate the body's stress response, and it can also help reduce fatigue, changes in appetite, and depression.

- **MAGNESIUM** works great alongside $B_6$ to help with cramps, fluid retention, headaches, and sleep. I recommend taking around 400 mg (in one dose before bed, or divided doses in the morning and evening). There are various forms, including glycinate, which doesn't affect digestion; citrate, which can loosen stools; threonate, which is great for brain function; and malate, which is great for sleep.

- **OMEGA-3 FATTY ACIDS** (2 to 4 grams a day) can help reduce cramps and other PMS symptoms. They act as phenomenal anti-inflammatories. It's important to find a high-quality source; I prefer pharmaceutical-grade omega-3s.

- **TURMERIC** reduces inflammation and can help with period pain. I recommend formulations with curcumin (1,000 mg), which is the active constituent of turmeric, and BioPerine (20 mg), which is a derivative of black pepper that can make curcumin more bioavailable.

- **VITAMIN D** is another important anti-inflammatory to take daily. I recommend 5,000 IU, but regularly testing your levels can keep you in the optimal range (50–80 ng/mL).

- **VITAMIN $B_6$** (25–50 mg) can be incredibly useful for both managing stress and also PMS symptoms, including moodiness, irritability, forgetfulness, bloating, and anxiety. It can also help your body produce more progesterone, which is helpful for women with estrogen dominance.

- **MOOD BOOSTERS.** I've found that saffron, SAM-e (400 mg), Zembrin (25 mg), or 5-HTP (100 mg) supplements help stabilize PMS moodiness. You don't need to take them together—try one at a time and see which one works best for you.

still growing and have high energy capacity, but they will really thrive if they get these calories from high-quality whole foods (which is not always the first choice of teens!).

There is so much pressure on young women to succeed these days. When you're going through puberty, your goals should be to be healthy, enjoy your life, and discover who you are and what you care about. Puberty can be an intense and confusing time because it's a rapid growth phase. It's important that young women give their bodies the nutrients they need rather than starving themselves, trying to fit into a certain clothing size. Fitness should be all about fun and the good feeling of moving their bodies, rather than focusing on attaining a certain physique.

### TEENS AND EARLY TWENTIES: DEVELOP GOOD HABITS NOW

Once girls get to high school, it's important for them to focus on continuing to build a healthy relationship to their bodies. Often this is when they start experimenting sexually, so if you are a parent to a teen or twentysomething, I urge you to discuss these subjects openly with your daughter. If you are in your twenties yourself, now is the time to learn safe sex habits.

Healthy eating and exercise habits teens develop now will be much easier to maintain later. I'm pretty sure I had problems with blood sugar metabolism when I was in high school and this played a role in how angry I was as a teenager. I was overloading my liver and taxing my pancreas with wild swings of insulin from junk food and processed foods. I wish I'd known then that dairy and refined sugar spiked insulin and made acne worse.

Another concern for teens as well as female athletes is not getting enough calories to support energy output. There is a serious condition that used to be called the female athlete triad[2] because it generally included three issues: disordered eating, amenorrhea (cessation

## PCOS

A lot of young women—as many as five million in the U.S.[3]—suffer from polycystic ovary syndrome (PCOS), which may go undiagnosed for years. This disease is characterized by high insulin levels that cause dysfunction in the ovaries, adrenals, and pituitary glands,[4] and many of the conditions that come along with that, including acne, depression, obesity, hormone imbalance causing irregular menstruation, and high cholesterol.

Elevated insulin stimulates the ovaries to make male hormones that disrupt fertility and menstrual regularity, and women with PCOS often have oligomenorrhea (infrequent menstrual periods, meaning less than six to eight per year). PCOS is highly correlated to metabolic disease—more than half of women with PCOS develop diabetes by the time they reach age forty. It's the most common cause of infertility in the United States, and it's considered a "multisystem reproductive metabolic disorder."[5]

One intervention for PCOS is a low-glycemic diet, which seems to work well for improving blood sugar and insulin control. Low-glycemic foods are low in refined carbohydrates and sugar, and higher in fiber and fat, which help to slow the release of sugar into the blood. A ketogenic diet—high in fat, low in carbs—may also help if you follow it periodically.

If you suspect you may have PCOS, I recommend seeing a functional medicine doctor versed in hormone health and asking to have your fasting insulin, fasting glucose, FSH, prolactin, free and total testosterone, TSH, IGF-1, and free T4 measured. PCOS is treatable, and you don't have to suffer.

of periods), and osteoporosis, due to the loss of bone mineral density caused by insufficient nutrition. Women who suffered from this condition were often participating in sports where being thin was considered desirable. This is now more commonly known as relative energy deficiency in sport, or RED-S, and the definition has expanded to refer to a syndrome that may include impaired menstrual function, bone health issues, protein synthesis issues, problems with metabolic rate, and cardiovascular health problems, all due to relative deficiency of energy or nutrition.[6] It's usually a result of an intentionally or unintentionally low-energy diet, with or without excessive exercise.

I'm mentioning this here because I know many women in their teens, twenties, and thirties who embark on biohacking journeys and stress their bodies to the point of nutrient deprivation. I've seen multiple women who's periods have stopped because of biohacking too intensely without proper calorie intake. This can cause insufficient bone mineral density, which can cause lifelong problems. What can you do to avoid this? You must make sure you are eating enough calories to meet your body's energy demands. Remember, the goal is to increase your energy potential! Undereating can lead to an energy availability (EA) deficit, which is the opposite of charging your batteries.

If you are very active or are a parent or mentor to a very active young woman, I suggest using the formula below to get a better sense of your or her EA:

EA = (total energy consumed [calories in] − total energy expended during exercise [calories out]) / kg of fat-free mass

To get your fat-free mass:

Fat-free mass = weight in kg − (body fat % x weight in kg)

To get your body fat percentage, use a smart scale that estimates this, or use an online body fat calculator. Or you can have a professional test done with body fat calipers or hydrodensitometry (this is an underwater measurement and is highly accurate).

Let's look at an example. A woman who weighs 140 pounds, or 63 kilograms, who has 20 percent body fat, works out and burns 500 calories. Her fat-free mass = 63 − (0.20 x 63) = 50. If she consumes:

1,200 calories, her EA = (1200 − 500) / 50 = 14 kcal per kg of fat-free mass per day

2,000 calories, her EA = (2,000–500) / 50 = 30 kcal per kg of fat-free
mass per day

2,700 calories, her EA = (2,750 - 500) / 50 = 45 kcal per kg of fat-free
mass per day

Having an energy availability of <30 kcal/kg of FFM means you've
got clinical low energy availability (LEA) that will impair health and
performance. Having an EA of 30–45 in women (30–40 in men) is
considered subclinical LEA, but may be tolerated during a period of
weight loss. Having an EA of >45 (>40 for men) is considered optimal
EA for weight maintenance.

I spent way too many years of my youth starving myself to fit an ideal
of perfection that was never reachable nor healthy. I see this behavior in
young women and their labs reflect profound undernourishment, which
is deeply troubling. If you are young, the best ways to lay the foundation
for metabolic health are to learn to lift weights, avoid being sedentary,
enjoy physical fitness, and *eat enough* for your demands. Undereating to
the point of RED-S deranges your metabolism, creates anxiety, causes
blood sugar imbalances, alters bone density (which can lead to early onset osteoporosis later in life), and contributes to hormonal dysfunction
(which can lead to low libido and fertility problems).

## LATE TWENTIES AND THIRTIES: MAKE FERTILITY DECISIONS

Even if you don't plan to have children, it's important to start monitoring your hormones in this life stage. One common issue women
face during their fertile years is estrogen dominance. Left unchecked,
it can increase your risk of breast cancer and other hormone-sensitive
cancers. Signs of estrogen dominance include:

- Irregular periods
- Heavy or long periods

- Clots in your menstrual blood
- Fibrocystic breasts or sore breasts before your period
- Weight gain, especially in your hips, thighs, and midsection
- Difficulty losing weight
- Fibroids, polyps, or growths in the uterus
- Endometriosis
- Insomnia
- Depression/anxiety/irritability
- Low libido
- Fatigue
- Problems conceiving
- PMS symptoms that are very disruptive to your life

If you suspect you have estrogen dominance, it's a good idea to get your labs checked with a functional medicine doctor who can perform blood and urine hormone testing as well as cycle mapping. Resources for this are on my website.

Luteal phase progesterone is something you should also consider checking, especially if you are in your late thirties and suffer from PMS or fertility issues. This test will tell you if you have too little progesterone, which can cause estrogen dominance symptoms. Progesterone deficiency can be managed with supplements or low-dose bio-identical progesterone replacement (but it's best to get a functional doctor to test your numbers and determine your best course of treatment).

Too much body fat can contribute to estrogen dominance, so knowing your body fat percentage can clue you in to whether this could be a problem. Estrogen dominance can also cause weight gain, especially around the belly, butt, hips, and thighs, which can lead to more estrogen dominance. Unfortunately, estrogen dominance can make weight loss problematic, which is why it is helpful to first find out what your hormone imbalance is with labs before you attempt weight loss.

## ESTROGEN DOMINANCE PROTOCOL

This protocol has two parts: dietary changes and supplement recommendations.

### Eating to Reduce Estrogen Dominance

• **BE STRICT ABOUT SUGAR.** This may be one of the most important things you can do to avoid breast cancer, because excess insulin puts your body into a growth state and high insulin can increase estrogen.

• **AVOID EXCESSIVE CONVENTIONAL MEAT AND DAIRY.** Good protein sources include fish, lean poultry, beans, nuts, and eggs.

• **GO GREEN.** Make sure you have filtered water and your food is organic. Aim for the highest-quality sources of lean meat, specifically grass fed/pasture raised. Increase your intake of fish, but be careful about mercury levels, as mercury is a COMT (catechol-O-methyltransferase) inhibitor, and COMT is an enzyme that metabolizes estrogen.

• **INCREASE INTAKE OF FIBROUS VEGETABLES,** which help clear estrogen through the stool and prevent its reabsorption into the body. Cruciferous veggies like broccoli, cauliflower, and cabbage are extra great for helping detox the liver.

• **INCREASE INTAKE OF COLORFUL VEGETABLES,** which provide antioxidants that help neutralize the more toxic estrogens (especially 4-hydroxy estrogens) the body produces.

• **INCREASE INTAKE OF FERMENTED FOODS.** Bad gut flora will cause too much estrogen to be reabsorbed rather than excreted, creating more risk for estrogen dominance and breast cancer. Make sure to feed your gut with fermented foods like yogurt, kimchi, kefir, and tempeh, or take probiotics.

• **LIMIT CAFFEINE** because caffeine and estrogen compete for clearance by the liver.

- **LIMIT ALCOHOL,** which can increase toxic types of estrogen due to reduced clearance by the liver. One glass of wine a day increases the risk of breast cancer by 40 percent.[7] At the most, drink one glass three times a week.

- **AIM FOR 35 GRAMS OF FIBER PER DAY,** to improve gut health and clear excess estrogen from the body.

- **MAKE SMOOTHIES** to help with hormone balance: Drink a daily smoothie with collagen or bone broth protein powder instead of whey protein for more stable insulin; add fiber like acacia fiber, chia, and flax; and add half a tablespoon of maca. One or two tablespoons of flaxseed a day is particularly helpful because flaxseeds are rich in lignans, which act as weak phytoestrogens that compete with your own estrogen in binding to estrogen receptors. Using flaxseed from the first day of your period until the first day of ovulation, around day fourteen, can also help to reduce symptoms of estrogen dominance.

### Biohack Estrogen Dominance with Supplements

Along with the baseline supplements vitamins D, $B_{12}$, and $B_6$; folate; and omega-3s, these additional supplements may help ease symptoms of too much estrogen:

- **MAGNESIUM** (400 mg a day) promotes healthy estrogen clearance by support- ing the COMT enzyme in the liver.

- **CALCIUM D-GLUCARATE** (500 mg) has been shown to help regulate excess estrogen levels.

- **DIM** (diindolylmethane, 100–200 mg) supports estrogen balance by increasing beneficial 2-hydroxy estrogens and reducing the unwanted 16-hydroxy variety. (Have your labs checked to see if you really need it before taking this.)

- **MILK THISTLE.** This is one of the most well-known liver-supporting nutrients (dosing ranges from 1,000 mg of pure herb to 150–250 mg of the extract).

Be careful of the following supplements that are the targets of COMT: quercetin, rutin, luteolin, EGCG, catechins, epicatechins, fisetin, and ferulic acid. Too much of these and your estrogen levels will rise. It's best to know your COMT status before taking these (you can find yours with data from basic genetic testing).

I had a client with the BRCA mutation (a genetic mutation that increases the risk of breast cancer). Along with extensive yearly imaging tests to catch any sign of cancer early, I also suggested lifestyle changes that could reduce her risk of excess estrogen buildup in her body. These changes can help anyone who is experiencing estrogen dominance. This is my estrogen dominance protocol.

### FORTIES: PREP FOR PERIMENOPAUSE

Throughout most of your forties, you may find you are coasting along feeling great, at the height of your career, and enjoying your family and (if you have them) children. Then, as you near the end of your forties, you will likely begin to experience the hormonal fluctuations of early perimenopause.

The beginning of perimenopause is marked by estrogen dominance, as progesterone is the first hormone to fall, and the ratio of progesterone and estrogen is important for hormonal balance. Perimenopausal women are also often estrogen deficient, which means that even though they have symptoms of estrogen dominance due to relative progesterone deficiency, their estrogen levels are declining. You can get a better idea of your hormone levels using urine hormone tracking (especially cycle mapping). A good functional doctor or naturopath can walk you through options like progesterone replacement to ease some of your symptoms.

As your estrogen gradually decreases throughout your late forties and into your early fifties, it's important to maintain your fitness (or start it up again), as less estrogen means lower bone density. Less estrogen can also lead to more insulin resistance and degradation of muscle, so this is the time of life when your carbohydrate needs go down and your protein needs go up. Choose more slowly metabolized, fibrous carbs and at least 40 grams of protein post-exercise.

Fasting-mimicking diets can be very beneficial during this stage

of life (such as the low-calorie five-day fasting program developed by
Dr. Valter Longo based on decades of research[8]). While the fasting-
mimicking diet is less extreme than fasting, it's important to listen to
your body. If you are under stress, don't fast.

## FIFTY TO SIXTY-FIVE: TRANSITION TO THE NEXT STAGE OF LIFE

Most women enter menopause sometime during this life stage. While
everyone's story is unique, the average age of menopause in the U.S.
is fifty-one. Menopause occurs on the day you have gone for an entire year without having a period[9]—everything after that is technically
postmenopause (although people generally refer to the years surrounding this day as "menopause" or as "being in menopause"). By sixty-five,
most women have experienced this full transition.

After menopause, you may find you achieve a new level of calm and
self-possession, and that can feel great. However, your body needs more
maintenance now, and that's important if you want to maintain your
healthspan for another few decades.

This is the time to start thinking about hormone replacement. If
you decide to go this route, it's better to start sooner rather than later,
to ease the transition and preempt the imbalance, rather than waiting
until your body has completely changed. Of course, hormone replacement isn't for everyone, especially if you are at high risk for breast
cancer, as hormone replacement therapy can increase breast cancer
risk. It's important to know that in a woman diagnosed with breast
cancer, hormone replacement is considered contraindicated. This must
be a carefully weighed decision between each woman and her care team.

As we get older, estrogen drops, which can cause vaginal dryness
and atrophy. Some women use vaginal estrogen cream to address vaginal dryness issues, but it's important to know that this form of estrogen
won't likely help with bone, heart, or brain health, just vaginal health.
Not only do estrogen and progesterone decline with age, but so does

testosterone, and this can tank your libido. (I have even seen low testosterone in women in their twenties, likely due to hormone-disrupting agents in the environment.) It's not uncommon for functional medicine doctors to prescribe low-dose topical bioidentical testosterone cream from a compounding pharmacy to boost libido for patients who are deficient.

This is also a time of life when we start to consider issues of neurological decline, and new research suggests there could be a link between estrogen deficiency and dementia. Estrogen replacement therapy seems to be more promising for helping mitigate dementia risk if it's started at menopause. The research suggests that waiting five years past menopause and then starting hormone replacement doesn't seem to be as helpful and may increase the risk of dementia.

After menopause, you are less insulin sensitive, and eating too many refined carbohydrates can cause weight gain and blood sugar instability. This is the time to focus on limiting growth and monitoring for unrestrained weight gain. You have less human growth factor, so your body has a greater tolerance for fasting and calorie restriction, which can be very beneficial, although of course you still need plenty of nutrient-dense foods.

Since you have very little estrogen, progesterone, and testosterone now, your body has a hard time increasing your muscle mass. I advise women in this life stage to lift heavy weights with fewer reps. This will help to maintain muscle and avoid frailty. Plyometrics (like jumping or exercises that use jumping motions) are great for strengthening bones and preserving power and speed. If you have arthritis in your joints, you might want to work with a trainer who knows how to provide you with weight-bearing exercises that are safe for your joints.

This is also a time to get serious about regular screening for health risks. All women over fifty should be getting screened for hypertension. Blood pressure tends to rise with age and is a major risk factor for heart disease. Other issues to begin screening for now, if you aren't already, are high cholesterol, breast cancer, colon cancer, cervical cancer, osteoporosis, obesity, alcohol use, depression, preventive aspirin in some cases (ask your doctor whether this is right for you), and vaccinations, when relevant. Go to your doctor once a year and get these tests done. Insurance will typically cover it.

## SIXTY-FIVE PLUS: STAY MOBILE, STAY FUELED, STAY CONNECTED

Your "menstrual" days are over, but you can still enjoy many vital years ahead if you're protecting your health. If you want to enjoy robust mental and physical health over the age of sixty-five, it's critical that you stay active and engaged in the world around you. You need to keep moving, keep exercising, and eat a nutrient-dense diet. One of the best things you can do for your mind is to exercise and keep learning, preferably at the same time. The more we engage in movement activities that challenge our minds, the more we can grow new neural connections and remain nimble and strong.

People often become interested in the secrets of longevity at this age. Avoiding chronic disease is critical to enjoying a long lifespan, and the more information we have about our health, the more able we are to make the kinds of changes that can help us live well for as long as possible.

The more you measure, understand, and track, the more you can take control of your body and your health risks. I started getting full-body MRIs at age thirty-six because I want to stay ahead of my health risks. You can stay ahead of your risks too, even if it's just checking your hormones a couple of times a year to see what your levels look like and adapting your lifestyle and habits to the needs of your current life stage.

HORMONE BIOHACKS IN THIS CHAPTER

- Track your cycle and the moon cycle to see if they match up.

- Test whether spending more time outside affects your cycle timing.

- Exercise to reduce cramps during your menstrual cycle.

- During the first week of your cycle, eat more foods rich in iron, vitamin C, and anti-inflammatory compounds, and take vitamin D.

- On days seven to thirteen of your cycle, push yourself at the gym, brainstorm new projects, and enjoy your creativity.

- On days thirteen to fifteen of your cycle, when ovulation occurs, be social, exercise moderately, and eat more fiber.

- On days fifteen to twenty-three of your cycle, plan projects, reflect, and don't push personal bests in the gym. Drink more water and take electrolytes if you are exercising a lot.

- On days twenty-four to twenty-eight, notice if you have any PMS symptoms and take PMS supplements if necessary like calcium, magnesium, omega-3s, turmeric, vitamin D, and vitamin $B_6$. Finish projects and reflect on your previous month. Do gentle, practice exercises like yoga and Pilates; and feed your cravings with healthy whole food.

- If you are an athlete or you're underweight, calculate your energy availability to determine how much to eat to avoid low energy availability or RED-S.

- In your twenties and thirties, assess fertility with hormone testing.

- If you have estrogen dominance, try my estrogen dominance protocol.

- Hack estrogen dominance with magnesium, calcium D-glucarate, DIM, and milk thistle.

- Fast more, or try the fasting-mimicking diet, in your forties.

- Test your hormones in your forties for signs of perimenopause.

- Track your cycle so you know when you have gone for one full year without a period and have officially achieved menopause.

- Talk to your doctor about whether HRT is right for you.

- Keep your brain healthy in your forties, fifties, and sixties with exercise and learning, and get enough protein.

# CHAPTER 13

# Biohacking Your Sexual Spark

Sex essence is the source of all energy available for creative and thinking processes (shien).

—Mantak Chia

As women, our sexuality is one of our greatest sources of power. It is a wellspring of energy that we can tap into if we learn how to sense and integrate it into the entirety of our being and our very existence. Cultivating our sexual energy and harnessing it for our pleasure and our partner's pleasure can make life extraordinarily beautiful. Sexual energy can be channeled into creative pursuits and can fuel our purpose in life.

Unfortunately, many people are simply out of touch with their sexual energy. Often our responsibilities take priority, and we forget how important pleasure is to living a good life. Sex can be fun and beautiful and an integral part of life and reproduction, but for many people it's awkward and uncomfortable. The only way to figure all of this out and develop a healthy, flourishing sex life is to be comfortable talking about it. How do we get there?

Women can feel empowered to communicate what they want and don't want. Men can learn to respect women's boundaries, listen, and understand that they don't know everything about a woman's body. Women often grow up with the idea that sex is something you do to please men, and there's not a lot of discussion around female pleasure, especially with younger women. This has resulted in generations of women who aren't comfortable acknowledging their sexual needs.

Now we're facing the fallout of this approach, with many women realizing that some past sexual interactions were not what they wanted, ranging on a spectrum from mild displeasure to devastating trauma. These have become issues that contribute to chronic stress and can compromise sexual satisfaction. What's worse, one in sixteen women's first sexual experience was nonconsensual, and according to the CDC, one in five women has been raped, one in four women was sexually abused as a child, and one in three women will be sexually assaulted in her lifetime. Sexual trauma can lead to sexual dysfunction, relationship dysfunction, and mental and physical health problems.

If you have a history of trauma, if your body gets triggered during sex, you may find that you can't communicate because you freeze. This is a polyvagal response that causes the body to become immobile and is a reason why people often freeze when they are in a fearful situation. I believe this may be why women with a history of sexual trauma have a higher risk of repeated trauma. This is part of the reason why I am on a mission to help women be more open to talking about sex and articulating their boundaries before getting into a situation that can be unpleasant at best and potentially traumatic. For more information, go to my website, where you'll find a list of questions for helping both women and men communicate with each other before they have sex to create physical and psychological safety.

## Hack Your Way to Better Sex

There are a lot of ways to improve the sexual experience for women, but at the core is the concept of safety. To be able to surrender to pleasure, you have to feel safe. Many women are still very much afraid of fully letting go during sex, and understandably. Feeling safe during sex may mean healing trauma first. For me, it wasn't until I started working on addressing past trauma that I was able to have powerful relationships that opened me up to what sex could really be.

Another part of being able to surrender to pleasure is getting out of your mind and into your body. I personally think that having really good sex with a partner begins with first knowing how to connect to yourself and how to connect to your own pleasure. If you don't know how to orgasm on your own, it's going to be challenging for somebody else to help you orgasm. I recommend educating yourself about different ways to orgasm, and also not being super attached to the outcome of sex, especially if you have trouble with orgasms. Being able to orgasm is like strengthening a muscle. You have to practice. Self-pleasure and

### HACKING YOUR ORGASMS

There is an ancient Taoist breathing technique called the microcosmic orbit that you can read about in the classic texts *Taoist Secrets of Love: Cultivating Male Sexual Energy* and *Healing Love Through the Tao: Cultivating Female Sexual Energy* by Mantak Chia. This technique involves breathing in and holding your pelvic diaphragm at the base of your pelvis up as you bring the diaphragm at the base of your lungs down, expanding your abdomen. Hold on to this energy, and then when you're having sex, you breathe it out, pushing the energy into the other person. It can be an amazing energetic exchange and it can work for genital sex, oral sex, or manual stimulation. By using this breathing technique and visualizing the circular orbit of the breath coming in and being pushed back out, you can dramatically improve the quality of sex and your orgasms. Bringing in your pelvic floor and holding it like that also trains your pelvic floor and strengthens your orgasm.

Kegels (intentionally contracting the muscles of your pelvic floor, including those around your clitoris) are another way to improve orgasms. I do Kegels all the time. The more you strengthen your pelvic floor, the more powerful your orgasms will be. Kegels are also important for women who have weaker pelvic floors from pregnancy and childbirth.

showing someone else how to pleasure you can significantly increase your pleasure during sex. That goes back to communication.

One small obstacle that gets in the way of pleasure is forgetting to breathe. Especially during the arousal phase, it's important to keep breathing and to make sure that you're using your breath to move your energy throughout your body. This will help your body relax as much as possible. We tend to tense up during sex, but letting yourself completely relax and then letting your partner help you become aroused can open the door to a more intense experience.

## When Arousal Is Difficult

Some women can be spontaneously aroused, but others need some time, and some women have problems getting aroused at all. To enjoy sex, you have to have a sex drive, and the sex drive is driven by testosterone and estrogen. If you suffer from problems with arousal and desire, you might want to get your testosterone level checked. Pretty much every time I've had a patient who had no interest in sex, we discovered she was deficient in testosterone, estrogen, or both. That's the first step to dealing with arousal issues—if you have a hormone deficiency, arousal will be biochemically problematic.

But there are also psychological barriers to arousal, from feeling insecure to feeling unsafe. One of the unfortunate side effects of long-term relationships, especially for women, is that the combination of the institution of marriage, the familiarity of living with a partner, and the desexualization of roles while raising children can lead to declines in sexual desire.[1] With the burdens of work and focus on caring for children, romance can wane, the relationship may take a backseat, and sex can become infrequent.

Reduced sexual desire can in turn threaten the relationship, as lack of sex leads to decreased intimacy, feelings of resentment, infidelity, and even divorce. But the most common impact of low desire on relationships is feeling "less connectedness" with one's partner.[2] For couples, that essential lack of connection can contribute to lack of sex, and lack of sex can worsen connection. Psychedelics and entactogens (love drugs) have a long history of use in the context of sexuality and are being studied for their potential to improve physical and emotional intimacy between long-term partners. They are also being studied as a possible solution for sexual dysfunction in men and women, which is often secondary to relationship problems, mood disorders, or trauma.

While reviewing the medical literature on sexual trauma, I discovered it can cause PTSD in 30 percent of women, and in 60 to 80 percent of women, it can lead to dysfunction. I personally experienced profound healing of multiple sexual dysfunctions secondary to sexual trauma using MDMA with a partner. Some women who've experienced sexual trauma can have orgasms alone, but they can't orgasm with a partner. The trauma is with them, like a box in the corner, and they don't want to open that box because they are afraid of not being able to handle what will come out. But in fact, it's the opening of the box and the moving through the trauma that can enable them to open up to a sexual partner. I recommend first working on trauma with a therapist, who can help you process that trauma in an environment that feels safe. A big piece of this is first lifting any shame you have about it.

At its core, good, pleasurable sex requires feelings of safety and trust, and the ability to get to a place where you can feel vulnerable with someone else. That may take some work, so no need to be in a hurry to jump into bed. Wait until you're ready.

## The Pros and Cons of Hormonal Birth Control

We all know what sex can lead to, and if you don't want to get pregnant now (or ever), at some point you're going to need to use birth control.

Birth control is one of the original biohacks, since sex is one of the original acts and pregnancy is one of the original inevitabilities. But pregnancy prevention isn't the only reason women go on birth control. One of the benefits many women experience on hormonal birth control is a reduction of PMS symptoms. This is a fix, but it's not a solution. I encourage my patients to investigate the cause of their symptoms rather than sweeping them under the rug with birth control. When you spend most of your adult life on hormonal birth control, you never really get to understand your cycles. Hormonal issues are suppressed while you're on birth control; if you go off your birth control, those problems will probably surface, but that gives you the chance to solve them while you are still young.

Most women do not realize that hormonal birth control is considered a class 1 carcinogen and that it increases your risk for heart attack, stroke, blood clots, and liver tumors. You may decide it's for you, but make that choice with knowledge.

## Fertility Challenges

When pregnancy is what you want, you may be thinking about your current or future fertility. For some women who wish to conceive, getting pregnant comes easily, but it's very common to face fertility challenges. Like so many other things, fertility can come down to mitochondrial health. It's the woman's mitochondria that are passed down to children. Without properly functioning mitochondria, the pregnancy may not carry. Mitochondria are responsible for powering life and the cell division required to turn a sperm and egg into a child. Optimal mitochondrial function will prolong fertility, plain and simple.

The first thing to do if you are trying to conceive and it doesn't seem to be working right away is to see a fertility specialist for testing.

Fertility labs can assess egg quantity and quality and detect ovulation. But you can support this with lifestyle. Here are some things you can do to maximize mitochondrial health and optimize fertility:

- GET ENOUGH NUTRIENTS. The following vitamins and minerals are crucial for optimal fertility:

  IRON. Iron deficiency has been linked to infertility, miscarriage, low birth weight, and preterm labor. Inadequate iron stores (having a ferritin level lower than 75 mcg/L) means you will be less likely to ovulate. Consider supplementation while you are getting to the root cause. We need around 18 mg a day, but when pregnant, this increases to 27 mg a day. Iron is important for energy metabolism because it helps red blood cells carry oxygen and transports it to the cells containing mitochondria, which burn the oxygen to provide energy to the body.

  COENZYME $Q_{10}$ IS IMPORTANT FOR MITOCHONDRIAL HEALTH. It's found in organ meats such as liver, kidney, and heart, as well as in beef, sardines, and mackerel. For plant-based folks, you can get it from vegetable sources including spinach, broccoli, and cauliflower. If you don't consume these regularly, you can supplement with 100 mg a day.

  VITAMIN C IS A POTENT ANTIOXIDANT THAT IS IMPORTANT FOR PROTECTING MITOCHONDRIA AGAINST OXIDATIVE INJURY. You can find this in citrus fruits, kiwis, and strawberries.

  FATS ARE IMPORTANT FOR FERTILITY. For women who eat a low-fat diet, it's important to know that your total cholesterol needs to be greater than 160 for optimal fertility.

  OMEGA-3S ARE CRUCIAL FOR BUILDING A BABY'S BRAIN. Fish is healthy because it contains omega-3s, but it does contain mercury.

Choose fish with lower mercury levels and get your mercury levels checked if you eat a lot of fish. If you don't eat fish, it's important to get your omega-3s checked, because if you are deficient, you should consider supplementing.

SELENIUM MAY ALSO HELP MAINTAIN THE HEALTH OF FOLLICULAR FLUID SURROUNDING WOMEN'S EGGS. A Brazil nut a day provides you with your recommended daily requirements. We need around 55 mcg daily for fertility and 65 mcg if we get pregnant.

- EAT FERTILITY-PROMOTING FOODS.

  BRIGHTLY COLORED VEGGIES AND FRUITS (ESPECIALLY THE RED ONES) ARE PARTICULARLY GOOD FOR FERTILITY AND MAY EVEN DELAY MENOPAUSE. These foods and other vegetables and fruits contain polyphenols and anti-inflammatory compounds. If you think you might not be getting enough, check your hs-CRP level, which can be an indicator of inflammation. If it's above 0.5, you probably need more produce in your diet.

  ACAI IS A GREAT ANTIOXIDANT-RICH FOOD YOU CAN TAKE THROUGH SUPPLEMENTS OR FIND IN YOUR FREEZER SECTION. For women who struggle getting enough produce, this can really help.

  EGGS ARE RICH IN CHOLINE, WHICH HELPS PREVENT BIRTH DE-FECTS. In general, the healthiest egg consumption seems to be one egg per day for optimal metabolic health.

  FULL-FAT DAIRY, CONDITIONALLY. Dairy has variable effects on women. In general, fat-free and low-fat dairy are suboptimal for fertility. Full-fat dairy may be helpful for underweight women with low hormone levels. In patients with autoimmunity or PCOS, con-sider limiting or eliminating dairy altogether for optimal fertility.

- **CHOOSE YOUR EXERCISE CAREFULLY.** Interval training and weight training can be amazing because they can boost mitochondrial biogenesis. Yoga is a fantastic option for boosting fertility because it can reduce stress and help with anxiety. On the other hand, chronic cardio is not optimal for fertility. The body adapts to chronic cardio by becoming more efficient with energy, and that can negatively impact fertility.

### FREEZING YOUR EGGS

If you want to have a baby someday, but you're just not sure when, you might be considering freezing your eggs. As I write this, I'm still in my fertile years and I'm planning on freezing my eggs. This will require injecting hormones (like human chorionic gonadotropin, follicle-stimulating hormone, human menopausal gonadotropin, gonadotropin-releasing hormone, etc.) or taking hormone-stimulating medications (e.g., Clomid) to induce what is known as "superovulation." The art of egg freezing is getting the most eggs you can without causing ovarian hyperstimulation syndrome, which can happen when your body makes too many eggs. Generally, the goal is to be able to extract between fifteen and thirty eggs. On the other hand, fewer than four eggs retrieved lowers pregnancy rates (and may necessitate another round of stimulation and harvesting in the future). After the eggs are stimulated, they need to be removed via a minor surgery in which your doctor uses an ultrasound-guided needle. Then your eggs are placed into cold storage and can be thawed and fertilized in the future. If that's not biohacking, I don't know what is.

The right age for egg freezing is up for debate. If you do it when you are young, your eggs will be less likely to have DNA damage. But some research suggests it's more cost-effective to do it around thirty-seven, when you are more likely to use them. For personalized advice, see a fertility specialist.

## Impairments to Fertility

Along with lifestyle choices that can increase fertility, there is a variety of influences that can impair fertility. If you want to have children, soon or just someday, it's important to be aware of the following factors:

- **FOODS WITH TRANS FATS.** This includes fast food, donuts, packaged pastries, and fried food. Studies have shown that 4 grams of trans fats a day is very bad for fertility.[3]

- **ALCOHOL.** In a large IVF study of 2,545 couples, women who drank four or more drinks per week were 16 percent less likely to carry a healthy child to term compared with those who drank less than four drinks per week (that's less than one drink per day). And the more a woman drank at the beginning of a cycle, the higher the rate of pregnancy loss. Another study of almost 3,000 couples showed that one serving of alcohol a month before IVF treatment tripled the risk of IVF failure; the risk was quadrupled if alcohol was consumed during the week of treatment.[4]

- **SOY.** Soy contains plant-derived estrogens called isoflavones. A 2022 study of Seventh-Day Adventists showed that the higher the isoflavone intake, the higher the risk of never having been pregnant.[5] If you are trying to conceive, aim for less than 40 grams of non-GMO, soy-based foods per day (one to three servings).

- **STIS OR PID.** STIs (sexually transmitted infections) like gonorrhea, ureaplasma, mycoplasma, and chlamydia can create pelvic inflammatory disease (PID), which can cause scarring of the fallopian tubes. Most doctors aren't testing for ureaplasma or mycoplasma so these can get missed. According to the CDC, tubal infertility occurs in 8 percent of women after just one episode of PID and can rise to as high as 40 percent after three episodes of PID.

- **LONG-TERM HORMONAL BIRTH CONTROL.** Birth control pills contain estrogen, which can alter the balance of thyroid hormones in the body. Estrogen increases thyroid binding proteins, which can reduce the amount of free thyroid hormones floating around. These are the active form of thyroid hormone, so for women on thyroid hormones and birth control pills, this can necessitate a higher dose of thyroid hormones. And if a woman goes off the pill, she may need to reduce the dose of how much thyroid hormone she takes.

## NOOTROPICS, CANNABIS, AND FERTILITY

Biohackers use nootropics, or "smart drugs," to hack the brain, boosting cognition, attention, and possibly intelligence, but at what price? One of the most popular nootropics, modafinil, is officially prescribed for narcolepsy, but it's often used by biohackers for cognitive enhancement. However, because modafinil increases liver enzyme activity in a way that can inhibit the liver's ability to break down contraceptives, it can make contraceptives less effective, resulting in an unintentional pregnancy. Since it could also cause birth defects when used by a pregnant woman, no one trying to get pregnant should be using modafinil for any reason.

Meanwhile, while marijuana/cannabis isn't exactly a nootropic, a 2016 study showed that marijuana could reduce female fertility because it disrupts the release of gonadotropin-releasing hormone from the hypothalamus,[6] which suppresses estrogen and progesterone production and may inhibit ovulation. The human body produces its own cannabinoids, and the researchers theorized that because fertility depends on the body's precisely regulating the endocannabinoid system, exogeneous cannabinoids from marijuana use could disrupt this balance and interfere with fertility. If you are trying to get pregnant, it's probably a good idea to lay off the marijuana use. A 2021 study showed that for each monthly cycle, women who had used cannabis and were trying to conceive were 41 percent less likely to conceive than nonusers.[7]

- **MOOD DISORDERS**. Studies suggest that mood disorders, in both the bipolar and unipolar spectrums, and anxiety may be associated with decreased fertility rates. Stress can tax the mitochondria, and we need healthy mitochondria for fertility.

- **CHRONIC HEALTH ISSUES**. If you have any chronic issues, like autoimmunity, anemia, low vitamin D, thyroid dysfunction, prediabetes or diabetes, fibroids, endometriosis, menstrual cycle irregularities (like cycles shorter than twenty-one days or longer than thirty-five days), absent periods secondary to undereating or obesity, painful periods, or PCOS, you may experience problems conceiving.

- **TOXIC BEAUTY AND CLEANING PRODUCTS**. Aim for clean products in your kitchen and your bathroom, and throughout your house, use cleaning supplies that are nontoxic. It's also a good idea to avoid nail salons while trying to get pregnant. Nail salons are filled with chemicals, including phthalates, which are known endocrine disruptors. Avoid Teflon and use of any plastics containing BPA. Better options for your kitchen are stainless steel and cast iron.

---

**SEX, BIRTH CONTROL, AND FERTILITY BIOHACKS IN THIS CHAPTER**

- Try the microcosmic orbit technique to strengthen your orgasms.

- Do regular Kegel exercises to strengthen your orgasms.

- Consider whether trauma is impacting your sexual pleasure and if you think it is, work with a therapist or counselor to process your trauma.

- Consider whether hormonal birth control is right for you.

- Enhance fertility by getting enough nutrients to support fertility, eating fertility-promoting food, and not overexercising to the point of stress.

- If you don't know when or if you will decide to have children but you are fertile now, consider freezing your eggs.

# CHAPTER 14

# Connection Is the Key to Longevity

*The key is to keep company only with people who uplift you. Whose presence calls forth your best.*

—Epictetus

I come from a large, tight-knit family, and I've always been a bit of a social butterfly, so connection with others has long been at the center of my life. But it wasn't until I started studying the impact of relationships on health while I was teaching at Stanford that I started to realize how essential human connection is for our long-term happiness, let alone our survival.

Social disconnection is a greater driver of disease than smoking, drinking, sedentary behavior, or obesity. And, as I have discovered, a lot of the reasons why people smoke, drink, and are obese or sedentary is because of problems with their relationships and their connections to community. Many of the people who struggle with addiction have a history of trauma or an attachment dysfunction from challenging early childhood or adult relationships. According to studies like the eighty-year Harvard study (on men), close personal relationships were the single greatest factor associated with long-term happiness.[1] So why is it that humans—who are wired as social animals—have lost touch with this essential pillar of health? And how can we get it back?

First, I think we need to fully appreciate the role that connection has long played for human beings. As you know, mitochondria evolved from primitive bacteria that were engulfed in a host organism and developed a symbiotic relationship. The bacteria harvested energy from the environment, expanding the organism's ability to survive. This was essentially the first relationship that helped life evolve. But what I only recently came to realize is that mitochondria evolved to become social organelles. What does this mean? Well, they act and behave in a lot of the same ways humans do in social networks—or it might be more accurate to say that we evolved to act and behave in a lot of the same ways mitochondria do!

Social behavior is conserved over multiple levels of life. Mitochondria form groups and act interdependently within them; they come together (through the process of fusion) to exchange information and distribute energy among the mitochondrial network, they exhibit synchronized behaviors (oscillating in unison to heartbeats and nerve cells' firing), they specialize to perform different functions in the cell, and they reproduce, breaking apart in a process called fission.[2]

We also evolved our social connections because it was adaptive to propagating life. We live together in shared environments. We merge with our partners during sexual contact and our babies during pregnancy. We communicate with each other with our voices, facial expressions, and body language, and through various technologies. We coordinate and synchronize our behaviors (think of team sports or group meetings in the office). We develop specialized skills and perform different social roles and have different professions so we can achieve collective goals. And, we give birth, creating new people.

After I became obsessed with mitochondria, one of the questions I asked myself was: If energy deficiency is the root of most chronic disease, then what is the root of energy deficiency? I realized that our relationship quality has a massive influence on our energy capacity. The quality of our relationships really determines the quality of our lives. On a behavioral level, when we struggle in our relationships, we often find ourselves exhausted and resorting to energy-draining forms of coping—eating junk food, binge-watching TV, addictions, and not moving our bodies. But there is also research that validates the impact of poor connections at the cellular level: studies show that chronic psychosocial stress can affect the number and quality of our mitochondria.[3] Different psychosocial stressors, including adverse childhood experiences, caregiving, stress, divorce, grief, and loss, affect the function of your cells.

Of course, the ability to connect with others starts with connecting with—and loving—ourselves. In my research on connection, I've found that one of the biggest barriers we have to loving others is not being able to truly love ourselves. It breaks my heart to hear stories from women about the trauma, abuse, neglect, family conflict, loss, perfectionism, toxic success, and self-harm they've endured—not to mention the burden of societal expectations for beauty and how this has affected their relationship to themselves. These problems degrade self-confidence and self-love. How can we expect to love ourselves when we live in a society that constantly tells us we aren't enough?

Even if you ignore everything else I have told you in this book, if you work on this one, single biohack—learning to love yourself—everything in your life will get easier. The path to self-love comes from self-discovery and working through all the barriers to truly looking in the mirror, really seeing ourselves, liking what we see, and loving who we are.

## The Paradox of Technology Use

Technology is amazing (and it can be an important ally in biohacking), but it has its dark side, including promoting unreal standards of what is considered attractive and hijacking our reward pathways, keeping us hunched over and unconscious of the anxiety this is causing.

Technology is here to stay, and I think we need a new approach to it if we are going to use it for our benefit and not let it completely run our lives.

Many doctors now routinely ask adolescents about their social media use (it's called the HEADSS screening) as part of a standard screening for issues with home life, education, activities, drug use, sexual activity, safety, suicide, and depression. An official "concerning response" for patients eleven years and older is spending over 120 minutes per day on social media, but I think that is a concerning amount of time on social media for anyone of any age. Smartphones and other devices and apps can track your screen use, to give you an idea of how much time you're spending looking at a screen.

There is a lot of research demonstrating mental health disturbances in teenagers who are heavy users of social media, including a growing number of studies associating smartphone use with student anxiety.[4] Gen Z, or those born between approximately 1997 and 2012, is the generation that is probably the most affected by technology because they are the first generation to have always had it, and studies of this generation have shown that they often experience serious psychological distress, major depression, and suicidal thoughts, and have more attempted suicides than any other generation, at a level far above millennials and older generations.[5] Instagram was released in 2010 and Snapchat in 2012 (just to give two examples), and research does suggest that the happiest Gen Z–ers are the ones who spend the least amount of time in front of screens. The "solution" of eliminating social media and internet use is obviously not going to happen, so we need to mitigate its negative effects.

One reason social media feels so addictive is because it creates a rush of dopamine that stimulates pleasure when you get a notification of some kind, then open up the message and discover the novelty of the information it contains. This quenches the desire you felt for connection, for a little while, until you get another ping. It's a dopaminergic loop, and that can become a behavioral addiction. It's not yet well studied enough to make it into the *DSM* (*Diagnostic and Statistical Manual of Mental Disorders*),[6] but I believe we will eventually see pathological internet use admitted to the *DSM*.

The benefits and risks of social media largely depend on the person and how they use it. If social media is having a negative effect on you—take some time to really consider whether it is—think about reducing your screen time. It seems pretty obvious that the more time anyone spends in front of screens, the less time they have for other, healthier experiences. In fact, some researchers say we are in the midst of a "cognition crisis." It's not a lack of information we struggle with. Instead, there is so much information coming at us all the time that our ability to perceive, integrate, and act on information has been compromised. It's believed this has led to hundreds of millions of people globally suffering from conditions associated with impaired cognition (e.g., depression, anxiety, dementia, autism, and ADHD, to name a few). Dr. Adam Gazzaley, a researcher at the University of California–San Francisco, has observed, "Constant engagement with technology interferes with the pursuit of other behaviors critical for maintaining a healthy mind such as nature exposure, physical movement, face-to-face contact, and restorative sleep. Its negative influence on empathy, compassion, cooperation, and social bonding are just beginning to be understood."[7]

Having experienced the consequences of too much stimulation and information overload myself, I've found a few things that have really worked for improving my focus and cognition, including monitoring and managing my technology use, keeping a regular meditation practice, using heart rate variability monitors to track stress and the efficacy of stress-management interventions, and mental fitness training like neurofeedback. Given the increasing role tech plays in our lives, I'm hopeful that in the future it will become commonplace to exercise our minds just as much as our bodies.

## Assessing Your Technology Use

Technology can create a barrier to human connection, an essential component of human health. How would you describe your relationship with technology? Think about these questions:

○ Do you use your phone as a stress reliever instead of taking a walk or deep breaths?

○ Do you purposely withdraw from difficult interactions by using your smartphone?

○ Does time seem to disappear when you're using your device?

○ Do you find yourself checking your phone while driving? Think seriously about how easily you could ruin your entire life with this habit.

○ When was the last time you posted unkind content or were targeted by someone else? How did it make you feel?

○ When was the last time you used your phone while having a meal with someone?

○ How often do you have the urge to photograph, document, and post everything? When was the last time you were just in the moment?

○ Do you get stressed while on your phone?

It's important to make time to unplug. Think about ways you can limit your phone time or create new habits around your technology use that result in more space for human connection.

## Connecting IRL

Although tech can help us feel connected to others who are far away, there simply is no replacement for in-person connection. Plenty of research has demonstrated that a network of social support promotes both physical and mental health.[8] Having more friends improves general health, including a lowered probability of obesity and depression,[9] while loneliness is a serious health risk.[10] Loneliness increases the risk of depression, cognitive decline, the progression of dementia, higher cortisol in the morning, higher blood pressure, illness, and premature death.[11] Social isolation increases stress-response pathways, and that can lead to mitochondrial and metabolic dysfunction. Over the long term, this could decrease your healthspan, as well as decreasing neurogenesis, while increasing inflammatory biology.

As we grow older, social activity remains critical for health and happiness. Research has shown that in people between the ages of sixty-seven and ninety-five, social activity is the strongest factor associated with happiness,[12] while older people with very little to no social interaction have higher suicide rates.[13] It's clear that humans just aren't built to be alone.

## Women Are Wired for Love

One of the many extraordinary qualities women possess: we are wired for love. We are oxytocin-dominant (oxytocin is a peptide hormone produced in the brain), and this gives us unbelievable gifts. We can have powerful orgasms, we can procreate, we can nurture, and we can build communities. All of these faces of being female are related to the magical hormone oxytocin. Men produce oxytocin as well, but they are vasopressin dominant, which means they are naturally wired for protection and defense.

## THE EVOLUTION OF SOCIAL CONNECTION

Loneliness is a primitive pain signal that we evolved because it would have encouraged us to move closer to our tribe. Being on the outskirts of a community would have put early humans at risk for being attacked by a wild animal or neighboring tribe. Moving closer would equate to greater safety. In primitive times, we would have lived in tribes or groups of people, and we would have supported each other. In many cultures around the world, there would be groups of women having children and helping each other raise the children, and groups of men who would go off hunting together, to provide food for the group. Everything people did, they did together, and in the service of the group and each other, rather than for themselves.

One way the world has changed, especially the modern Western world, is that "rugged individualism" is celebrated as a positive thing. In Western culture, people tend to act with self-interest. You find your own resources to support your very small immediate nuclear family. Today, even the immediate family is often fragmented, with children born to single parents, parents having to work multiple jobs to support their families, and rampant feelings of isolation, loneliness, and stress, even though we know that our relationships determine our level of well-being and influence our health. If we can remember how important social connection was for our early survival, we might begin to understand how essential it is for our survival now and into the future.

In primitive times, these social roles would have kept the species alive. In fact, it's hypothesized that we evolved oxytocin after vasopressin, enabling us to form tight, cohesive social groups. Oxytocin facilitates the experience of social reward. When we feel connected, calm, and safe with our trusted friends and family, that's oxytocin at work.

Oxytocin (along with dopamine, serotonin, and norepinephrine) helps facilitate our experience of love for a reason. Love is not just an emotion but a motivational force, just like hunger or thirst, that drives people toward one another to share information and resources and increase proximity between the sexes, which increases the probability of reproduction.[14] In fact, oxytocin is made in the part of the brain (the hypothalamus) that is responsible for the regulation of food intake, and it plays a crucial role in feeding and appetite.[15] Oxytocin promotes fat burning, weight loss, and insulin sensitivity independent of its effects on food intake. It helps reduce appetite and visceral fat.[16] It acts as both an anti-inflammatory and an antioxidant.[17] It also enhances wound healing, promotes bone health, and improves lipid and glucose metabolism. Basically, it protects our mitochondria and our metabolic health. This is part of the reason why positive social relationships are correlated with longevity. According to the brilliant scientist Sue Carter, oxytocin may actually be nature's medicine.[18]

But it gets better. Oxytocin also facilitates the birthing process, lactation, child-rearing and maternal behavior, growth of the neocortex in babies, the nurturing necessary for intellectual development, and the social sensitivity and attunement necessary for developing social behaviors. Oxytocin is the glue that enables pair bonding, parent-child bonds, familial bonds, and social bonds.[19] There's a theory that long-term pair bonds and family relationships facilitated the evolution of social intelligence and cooperative skills. Oxytocin is the hormone that made that happen.

Realizing how fundamental this neurochemistry was to life itself opened my eyes to why we are seeing so many diseases of despair in a society mired with social disconnection. When it comes to survival, love is just as important as food, and without it, humans fail to thrive. This is why lack of love and lack of social connection are so unbelievably detrimental to human health and predispose people to addiction, social conflicts, mental illness, and even obesity and metabolic diseases. Researchers believe that oxytocin's main role is to enable us to "facilitate stability in changing environments." This means our relationships actually determine our capacity to adapt to the challenges we face.

## Increasing Oxytocin for Better Connection and Health

The first step to boosting oxytocin production is to strengthen your social connections. This requires an investment of time and attention to others. Prioritize the people who matter to you by spending quality time with your family and your friends. Helping other people from the goodness of your heart is another way to do this, whether that may be volunteering in your community or helping out a friend who needs an important favor.

Second, take advantage of the oxytocin-boosting power of touch. Touch is an essential way babies bond with parents. (Did you know that just holding a baby releases oxytocin in your brain? Babies literally program you to bond to them.) The best research we have on touch is through studying children from orphanages. Children who don't receive enough physical touch are at an increased risk for experiencing various developmental delays. Touch is also a means of creating deeper social bonds. Lack of touch is likely one reason why isolation, loneliness, and rejection are associated with poor physical and psychological health.

In primitive times, a lack of human touch represented a legitimate safety threat, as it was dangerous to be separated from the group. Touch gives the sense that we are connected to others, and that makes us feel safe. I'm a huge believer in massage therapy as another way to biohack touch receptors. Even if you don't know the person, that skin contact is powerful. If you can't get a massage, even just softly stroking your own arm can induce calm in your nervous system.

Other ways to enhance oxytocin release aside from touch, positive social relationships, and positive in-person social connection are practicing gratitude, expressing appreciation for others, and exhibiting compassionate behavior toward other people. Emotional attunement to others also promotes a felt sense of safety. I learned the central tenants of Imago Therapy, which are mirroring, empathizing, and validating another's experience and discovered this is a great way not only to connect with another's emotional experiences, but also to resolve conflict by reestablishing psychological safety in challenging situations.

One of the most profound forms of oxytocin release, and the reason why sex is so potent in inducing romantic love and attachment, is orgasm. I have studied the work of many scientists who research love and discovered that the more we have sex with a person, the more our body releases the neurochemical signals of love. Dopamine gives us a sense of awe, ecstasy, euphoria, passion, and significance. Serotonin gives us a warm and fuzzy feeling and general sense of well-being in the presence of someone else. Norepinephrine can make us so obsessed with someone else that we forget to eat or can't sleep. In a lot of ways, developing the feelings of romantic love is like experiencing a physiological addiction to someone. Oxytocin is the glue that binds us together and creates the attachment of long-term love.

Researchers believe all drives, like hunger, thirst, sex, and love, involve dopamine pathways because the reward of pleasure ensures our innate biological needs are met.[20] Dopamine is thought to be central to sexual motivation because it enables focused attention on a single partner. Interest in other sexual partners falls away, especially during early romantic love and courtship.[21] This is biology's way of inducing an addiction to another person to ensure mate preference.[22]

On the flip side, when people have breakups or lose partners to accidents or illness, they may suffer from withdrawal symptoms, become clinically depressed, experience suppressed immunity, and even end up suicidal or harming others. When we fall madly in love with someone and have sex, touch them, and have orgasms with them regularly, we also start to get attached to them because of the hormone oxytocin. Scientists believe humans evolved romantic love as a "commitment device" that drives pair bonding, which predicts better survival of parents and offspring.[23] Researchers also posit that familial love evolved to keep the family intact, which enhances all members' survival. Part of the reason why loss of love is experienced so dramatically is that our social bonds are intimately tied to our survival and passing on our genes—the biological imperative. When this is threatened, we suffer immensely.

### OXYTOCIN AND THE PLACEBO RESPONSE

Oxytocin is probably a player in the placebo response—when a medicine or treatment works because you think it will—and is likely dependent on the warmth and trust of care providers. Those who inspire trust (make frequent eye contact, smile, engage in active listening, behave confidently and with interest) induce a sense of safety and the release of oxytocin in those they are caring for. When a mother kisses her child's boo-boo, she's using oxytocin as medicine to make them feel better. And that medicine works! How cool is that?

## The Energy of Love

Mother Teresa once said, "The greatest disease in the West today is not TB or leprosy; it is being unwanted, unloved, and uncared for. We can cure physical diseases with medicine, but the only cure for loneliness, despair, and hopelessness is love." Love is the final secret to extended healthspan, a long life, and fulfillment. It is the force that brings people together to create more life, more security, more vitality, and ultimately, more meaning. It is the divine and luminescent spark within us all. It is the deepest, most potent, most beautiful thing we all have in common.

This book defines health as the ability to adapt and thrive in the face of adversity, and yes, physical resilience does that, but so does love. Strength, power, and resilience mean little without love to animate and drive them. We need closeness and security to grow and flourish. The more we love, the less we fear. The more we love, the more fiercely we protect our loved ones. The more we let love lead our lives, the faster we heal and the more we crave life. The more we love, the more we *thrive*.

Life energy flows through our cells like circuitry, and even on a cellular level, our cells sense safety or danger and react appropriately. I believe underneath all life, the very fabric of the universe is a field of infinite intelligence, love, and beauty by which all creation springs forth into reality. When we tap into this divine energy, we learn to fully enjoy life. Sex becomes a transformative experience. Family becomes a purpose. Loving yourself becomes a sacred act. The more we nurture love within ourselves and our relationships, the more we become self-actualized and the more we can transcend our egos and live a life of service to humanity.

When we unlock the spark within each of us, by caring for our bodies and cultivating the life-force energy flowing through our mitochondria, we become capable of much more than we ever dreamed. We become capable of loving others, caring for others, elevating our communities, and understanding at the cellular level what life is for. The capacity we get from health and the love we cultivate within ourselves can transform existence and make the lives we live as full, ripe, and luminescent as they can be.

My friends, be radiant and light the world. The healthier you are, the more you glow. So go on. Get out there, come alive, and shine.

*Love,*
*Dr. Molly*

# Acknowledgments

I want to thank Eve Adamson, Alex Glass, and Gabrielle Mattson, who were instrumental in making this book happen; my publishing team at Harper Collins: Julie Will, Emma Kupor, Karen Rinaldi, Amanda Pritzker, Yelena Nesbit, Nikki Baldauf, and Robin Bilardello; my mother, father, and sisters, Nikki, Corinne, Alison, and Madison, who are my favorite people in the whole world; my friends, who have been such major supporters of my life and career, including Katrine Volynsky, Sarah Kaney, Tom Chi, David Pierce Jones, Todd Huffman, Robin Connelly, John Stanton, Celia Chen, Anthony Lemme, Gavriella Ravid, Robert Oliver, Ryan Bethencourt, Jonathan Yaffe, Brandilyn Brierley, Rebecca Jean Alonzi, Finn McKenna, Ian Mitchell, Dave Korunsky, Dave Morin, Lonnie Rae Kurlander, Megan Klimen, Daniel Schmachtenberger, James Schmachtenberger, Sanjiv Sidhu, Suki Mehr, Paris Rouzati, Anderson Pugash, Aneel Chima, Sarah Meyer Tapia, Michael Vassar, Terri Hinton, Alastair Trueger, Matthew Goodman, Matt Wiggins, Zach Bell, Bear Kittay, Max Marmer, Justin Boreta, Jeremy Gardner, Phaedra Randolph, Ben Metcalf, Dustin Robertson, Benjamin James Smith, Sumaya Kazi, Peter Barsoon, Perla Piergallini, Gil Penchina, Nicole Asarche, Chad Asarche, Dallas Hartwig, Rene Graham, Leemor Chandally, Noah Karesh, Stephanie Liu, Ø. Benum, Justin Shaffer, Graham

Pilger, Andrew Wilkinson, Mel Weinberger, Aaron Michael, John Michael Collins, Andrei Karkar, Paris Rouzati, Jivan Achreja, Jason Karp, Antoun Nabhan, James Beshara, Justin Boreta, William Chou, David Mehlman, Todd Baldree, Matt Ciociolo, Sylvia Benito, Peter Barsoom, Ryan Howard, Noa Kahner, Tatiana Strauss, Christian Edler, Dustin Robinson, Dominique Pitts, James Clement, Hindy Friedman, Bobby Brazen, Kiana Soleiman, Loana Karras, Justin Kahn, Penny Lane, Tammetrius Farmer, and Sharika Majeti; to Garrett Lisi, whose generosity enabled me to begin writing this book while I was staying at the Pacific Science Institute in Maui; to Todd Shipman who introduced me to PaleoFx, where I met Eve Adamson and Alex Glass; to Kathleen Sage, who gave me great legal advice; to Jonathan Jacobs, who helped me with the marketing; to Dr. Casey Means, Josh Clemente, and Sam Corcos of Levels and the JPTR team, who helped me tremendously with the book launch; to Jay Wiles, who helped me by teaching me more about HRV than anyone else; to Ben Gibson, who opened my eyes to the power of mitochondria; to Dave Asprey, for being such a massive inspiration; to the many doctors and academic professionals who have been friends and mentors during my journey, including Dr. Sue Carter, Dr. Stephen Porges, Dr. Ben Kaplan Singer, Dr. Stephanie Coleman, Dr. Stephanie Daniel, Dr. Jason Camm, Dr. Edward Rich, Dr. Maqbool Ali, Dr. Terry Brady, Sue Goldsteine, Dr. Irwin Goldstein, Dr. Barry Komisaruk, Dr. Ally Feduccia, Dr. Brian D. Earp, Dr. Helen Fisher, Dr. Saida Desilets, and Dr. Adam Gazzaley.

# How to Do an Elimination Diet

I recommend going on an elimination diet to every single one of my patients. This is a method for eliminating potentially allergenic as well as packaged and processed foods. An inflammatory diet can cause your body to overreact to many things. When you clean up your diet this way, you calm that reactivity, so you can get a better idea of what you *actually* react to and what your body can tolerate. At this point, you can slowly reintroduce the foods you like, to see how your body reacts. This will help you understand at a visceral level what's working and what's not working for you. Then, any necessary food restriction becomes about actually knowing what *feels* good, rather than about willpower.

The basics of an elimination diet are to eat a very simple, non-allergenic diet for at least four weeks, before reintroducing individual food groups to see how you react. (If you have an autoimmune disease, you can stay on this diet indefinitely, but most people will likely want to reintroduce some foods.) That means eliminating some of the most common irritants:

- Gluten
- Grains
- Legumes
- Corn

- Soy
- Dairy
- Added sweeteners, including artificial sweeteners
- Inflammatory oils: corn, soy, canola, sunflower, safflower, cottonseed, grapeseed, peanut
- Alcohol (Tough, but try. If you do drink, keep it gluten-free and no more than one or at maximum two drinks per week. Gluten-free liquors are rum, tequila, and potato vodka. Most wines and ciders are also gluten-free. No beer.)
- Coffee and caffeinated energy drinks (Also tough, but once you get over the first few foggy days, taking a caffeine break feels amazing.)
- Additives, like carrageenan, gums, and artificial flavors and colors
- Anything else you already know you are sensitive to (e.g., nuts, seeds, fish, and eggs sometimes bother people)

Eat only fresh grass-fed, pastured, or wild meat, poultry, and seafood; fresh vegetables and fruits; soaked and sprouted nuts and seeds (if you tolerate them); animal fats like lard and ghee; fruit oils like olive, avocado, and coconut oil; fresh pastured eggs (if you're not sensitive to them); very small amounts of natural sweeteners like honey and maple syrup; and lots of herbs and spices.

After your elimination period, you can begin to reintroduce foods. Do this systematically and carefully, with self-awareness, and focus on single foods, not combination foods like pizza or sandwiches, or you won't be able to isolate what's bothering you. Pay close attention to any symptoms you get after eating each reintroduced food, keeping a written record of what you are reintroducing and what symptoms recur (it's easy to forget—write it down). For example, you might try some milk or cheese after four to six weeks without dairy, then wait three days. If you notice a recurrence of symptoms, that's a sign that you are sensitive to dairy. If you feel fine, that means you may be able to eat dairy products without any problem, at least in small amounts.

An elimination diet helps you create a baseline for your nutrition. After that baseline, you can go on to tweak and hack your diet further, in terms of blood sugar, metabolic flexibility, and microbiome health.

For a more detailed explanation of my elimination diet protocol, expanded food lists, portion sizing, cooking instructions, and basic easy recipes for smoothies, salads, snacks, and my favorite cold green soup, go to my website. For a simplified elimination diet program, you can try Whole30 or the autoimmune Paleo diet (as described in the book *The Wahls Protocol*).

# Resources

There are many great resources out there that can expand your knowledge about health, mitochondria, and biohacking. I've mentioned some of these throughout the book, but there are far more than I could list, and so much to learn about your body, mind, and health. Here are some of my favorites, for further study:

*8 Steps to a Pain-Free Life* by Esther Gokhale

*The Big Leap* by Dr. Gay Hendricks

*Come As You Are* by Emily Nagoski

*The Complete Guide to Fasting* by Dr. Jason Fung

*Complex PTSD: From Surviving to Thriving* by Pete Walker

*Diagnosis and Treatment of Chronic Fatigue Syndrome and Myalgic Encephalitis: It's Mitochondria, not Hypochondria* by Dr. Sarah Myhill

*Do Less: A Revolutionary Approach to Time and Energy Management for Ambitious Women* by Kate Northrup

*Good Morning, I Love You* by Shauna Shapiro

*Healing Back Pain: The Mind-Body Connection* by John E. Sarno

*Letting Go* by David R. Hawkins

*Love Drugs* by Brian Earp and Julian Savulescu

*Roar* by Stacy Sims

*Self-Compassion* by Kristin Neff

*She Comes First: The Thinking Man's Guide to Pleasuring a Woman* by Ian Kerner

*Taoist Secrets of Love: Cultivating Male Sexual Energy* and *Healing Love Through the Tao: Cultivating Female Sexual Energy* by Mantak Chia

*Why We Get Sick* by Dr. Benjamin Bikman

# Notes

## Chapter 1: Energy Powers Life

1. Craig Becker and William Mcpeck, "Creating Positive Health: It's More Than Risk Reduction." *NWI White Paper*, December 11, 2013.

2. Francesca E. Duncan, Emily L. Que, Nan Zhang, et al., "The Zinc Spark Is an Inorganic Signature of Human Egg Activation," *Scientific Reports* 6 (2016), https://www.nature.com/articles/srep24737.

3. J. Graham Ruby, Kevin M. Wright, Kristin A. Rand, et al., "Estimates of the Heritability of Human Longevity Are Substantially Inflated Due to Assortative Mating," *Genetics* 210, no. 3 (2018), https://doi.org/10.1534/genetics.118.301613.

4. Michael Lustgarten, *Microbial Burden: A Major Cause of Aging and Age-Related Disease* (self-published ebook, 2016), https://www.amazon.com/Microbial-Burden-Major-Age-Related-Disease-ebook/dp/B01G48A88A.

5. "Deaths: Final Data for 2016," *National Vital Statistics Reports* 67, no. 5 (2018): 76.

6. Elizabeth Arias, Betzaida Tejada-Vera, Farida Ahmad, and Kenneth D. Kochanek, "Provisional Life Expectancy Estimates for 2020," *NVSS Vital Statistics Rapid Release,* report 15 (July 2021), https://www.cdc.gov/nchs/data/vsrr/vsrr015-508.pdf.

7. "Heart Disease and Stroke Cost America Nearly $1 Billion a Day in Medical Costs, Lost Productivity," CDC Foundation, April 29, 2015, https://www.cdcfoundation.org/pr/2015/heart-disease-and-stroke-cost-america-nearly-1-billion-day-medical-costs-lost-productivity.

8. "CDC Prevention Programs," American Heart Association, May 18, 2018, https://www.heart.org/en/get-involved/advocate/federal-priorities/cdc-prevention-programs.

9. Farhad Islami, Ann Goding Sauer, Kimberly D. Miller, et al., "Proportion and Number of Cancer Cases and Deaths Attributable to Potentially Modifiable Risk Factors in the United States," *CA: A Cancer Journal for Clinicians* 68, no. 1 (2018), https://doi.org/10.3322/caac.21440.

10. "National Diabetes Statistics Report," Centers for Disease Control and Prevention, January 7, 2022, https://www.cdc.gov/diabetes/library/features/diabetes-stat-report.html.

11. "Prediabetes—Your Chance to Prevent Type 2 Diabetes," Centers for Disease Control and Prevention, December 21, 2021, https://www.cdc.gov/diabetes/basics/prediabetes.html; "National Diabetes Statistics Report: Estimates of Diabetes and Its Burden in the United States," Centers for Disease Control and Prevention, January 18, 2022, https://www.cdc.gov/diabetes/data/statistics-report/index.html.

12. National Center for Chronic Disease Prevention and Health Promotion, Centers for Disease Control and Prevention, https://www.cdc.gov/chronicdisease/index.htm.

13. World Health Organization Constitution, https://www.who.int/about/governance/constitution.

14. M. Huber, M. Van Vliet, M. Giezenberg, et al., "Toward a 'Patient-Centred' Operationalization of the New Dynamic Concept of Health: A Mixed Methods Study," *BMJ Open* 6, no. 1 (2016), https://doi.org/10.1136/bmjopen-2015-010091.

15. "CMS: US Health Care Spending Will Reach $4T in 2020," *Advisory Board*, April 3, 2020, https://www.advisory.com/daily-briefing/2020/04/03/health-spending.

16. "Stress in America 2020: A National Mental Health Crisis," American Psychological Association, October 2020, https://www.apa.org/news/press/releases/stress/2020/report-october.

17. Pauline Anderson, "Physicians Experience Highest Suicide Rate of Any Profession," Medscape, May 7, 2018, https://www.medscape.com/viewarticle/896257; Centers for Disease Control and Prevention. "Supplementary Table 2: Male and Female Suicide Rates per 100,000 Civilian, Noninstitutionalized Working Persons Aged 16–64 Years for Major and Detailed Occupational Groups Meeting Reporting Criteria, National Violent Death Reporting System, Suicide Decedents (n = 15,779), 32 States, 2016," *Morbidity and Mortality Weekly Report* 69, no. 3 (2020), https://stacks.cdc.gov/view/cdc/84275.

18. Esther G. Gerrits, Heeln L. Lutgers, Nanne Kleefstra, et al., "Skin Autofluorescence: A Tool to Identify Type 2 Diabetic Patients at Risk for Developing Microvascular Complications," *Diabetes Care* 31, no. 3 (2008), https://doi.org/10.2337/dc07-1755.

19. Deepika Pandhi and Deepshikha Khanna, "Premature Graying of Hair," *Indian Journal of Dermatology, Venereology, and Leprology* 79, no. 5 (2013), https://doi.org/10.4103/0378-6323.116733.

## Chapter 2: Mitochondria: Your Cellular Batteries

1.  Rene Morad, "Defeating Diseases with Energy," Scientific American Custom Media, January 9, 2018, https://www.scientificamerican.com/custom-media/jnj-champions-of-science/defeating-diseases-with-energy/.

2.  Sanjeev K. Anand and Suresh K. Tikoo, "Viruses as Modulators of Mitochondrial Functions," *Advances in Virology 2013* (2013), https://www.hindawi.com/journals/av/2013/738794/.

3.  Nature Education, "Virus," Scitable: A Collaborative Learning Space for Science, 2014, https://www.nature.com/scitable/definition/virus-308/.

4.  Sean Holden, Rebeckah Maksoud, Natalie Eaton-Fitch, et al., "A Systematic Review of Mitochondrial Abnormalities in Myalgic Encephalomyelitis/Chronic Fatigue Syndrome/Systemic Exertion Intolerance Disease," *Journal of Translational Medicine* 18, no. 290 (2020), https://dx.doi.org/10.1186%2Fs12967-020-02452-3.

5.  W. M. H. Behan, I. A. K. More, and P. O. Behan, "Mitochondrial Abnormalities in the Post Viral Fatigue Syndrome," *Acta Neuropathologica* 83 (1991), https://doi.org/10.1007/bf00294431.

6.  "A Mitochondrial Etiology of Common Complex Diseases," UCLA CTSI, YouTube, May 23, 2017, https://www.youtube.com/watch?v=1aCHrHwm_AI.

7.  Yanping Li, An Pan, Dong G. Wang, Xiaoran Liu, et al., "Impact of Healthy Lifestyle Factors on Life Expectancies in the US Population," *Circulation* 138, no. 4 (2018), https://doi.org/10.1161/CIRCULATIONAHA.117.032047.

8.  Michael Ristow and Katherine Scheisser, "Mitohormesis: Promoting Health and Lifespan by Increased Levels of Reactive Oxygen Species (ROS)," *Dose-Response* 12, no. 2 (2014), https://dx.doi.org/10.2203%2Fdose-response.13-035.Ristow.

9.  Li et al., "Impact of Healthy Lifestyle Factors."

10. Richard L. Auten and Jonathan M. Davis, "Oxygen Toxicity and Reactive Oxygen Species: The Devil Is in the Details," *Pediatric Research* 66 (2009), https://www.nature.com/articles/pr2009174.

11. Caroline Hadley, "What Doesn't Kill You Makes You Stronger: A New Model for Risk Assessment May Not Only Revolutionize the Field of Toxicology, but Also Have Vast Implications for Risk Assessment," *EMBO Reports* 4, no. 10 (2008), https://doi.org/10.1038%2Fsj.embor.embor953; Anton Gartner and Alper Akay, "Stress Response: Anything That Doesn't Kill You Makes You Stronger," *Current Biology* 23, no. 22 (2013), https://doi.org/10.1016/j.cub.2013.09.036.

12. Ari Whitten, The Energy Blueprint, https://theenergyblueprint.com/.

13. Rhonda P. Patrick and Teresa L. Johnson. "Sauna Use as a Lifestyle Practice to Extend Healthspan." *Experimental Gerontology* 154 (October 15, 2021), https://doi.org/10.1016/j.exger.2021.111509.

14. Se-A Kim, Yu-Mi Less, Je-Yong Choi, David R. Jacobs Jr., and Duk-Hee Lee, "Evolutionarily Adapted Hormesis-Inducing Stressors Can Be a Practical Solution to Mitigate Harmful Effects of Chronic Exposure to Low Dose Chemical Mixtures," *Environmental Pollution* 233 (2018), https://doi.org/10.1016/j.envpol.2017.10.124.

15. Philip L. Hooper, Paul L. Hooper, and Laszlo Vigh, "Xenohormesis: Health Benefits from an Eon of Plant Stress Response Evolution," *Cell Stress and Chaperones* 15, no. 6 (2010), https://www.ncbi.nlm.nih.gov/pmc/articles/PMC3024065/.

## Chapter 3: The Quantified Self: Biohacking to Create Health

1. Stacy T. Sims, *Roar* (Rodale, 2016).

2. Karen Zraick and Sarah Mervosh, "That Sleep Tracker Could Make Your Insomnia Worse," *New York Times*, June 13, 2019, https://www.nytimes.com/2019/06/13/health/sleep-tracker-insomnia-orthosomnia.html.

3. "Find a Practitioner," Institute for Functional Medicine, https://www.ifm.org/find-a-practitioner/.

## Chapter 4: Movement Is Life's Energy Signal

1. Frank W. Booth, Christian K. Roberts, John P. Thyfault, et al., "Role of Inactivity in Chronic Diseases: Evolutionary Insight and Pathophysiological Mechanisms," *Physiological Reviews* 97, no. 4 (2017), https://doi.org/10.1152/physrev.00019.2016.

2. Centers for Disease Control and Prevention, "Physical Activity and Health: A Report of the Surgeon General," November 17, 1999, https://www.cdc.gov/nccdphp/sgr/adults.htm.

3. Booth, et al., "Role of Inactivity in Chronic Diseases."

4. Lin Yang, Chao Cao, Elizabeth D. Kanter, et al., "Trends in Sedentary Behavior Among the US Population, 2001–2016," *JAMA* 321, no. 16 (2019), https://doi.org/10.1001/jama.2019.3636.

5. University of North Carolina at Chapel Hill, "Only 12 Percent of American Adults Are Metabolically Healthy, Study Finds," ScienceDaily, November 28, 2018, https://www.sciencedaily.com/releases/2018/11/181128115045.htm.

6. David A. Raichlen and Gene E. Alexander, "Adaptive Capacity: An Evolutionary Neuroscience Model Linking Exercise, Cognition, and Brain Health," *Trends in Neurosciences* 40, no. 7 (2017), https://dx.doi.org/10.1016%2Fj.tins.2017.05.001.

7. Booth et al., "Role of Inactivity in Chronic Diseases."

8. Booth et al., "Role of Inactivity in Chronic Diseases."

9. Booth et al., "Role of Inactivity in Chronic Diseases."

10. Steven N. Blair, "Physical Inactivity: The Biggest Public Health Problem of the 21st Century," *British Journal of Sports Medicine* 43, no. 1 (2009), https://bjsm.bmj .com/content/43/1/1.

11. Ann Regina Lurati, "Health Issues and Injury Risks Associated with Prolonged Sitting and Sedentary Lifestyles," *Workplace Health and Safety* 66, no. 6 (2018), https://doi.org/10.1177/2165079917737558.

12. Booth et al., "Role of Inactivity in Chronic Diseases."

13. M. Neuhaus, E. G. Eakin, L. Straker, et al., "Reducing Occupational Sedentary Time: A Systematic Review and Meta-analysis of Evidence on Activity-Permissive Workstations," *Obesity Reviews* 15, no. 10 (2014), https://doi.org/10.1152/jappl physiol.00925.2005.

14. Neuhaus et al., "Reducing Occupational Sedentary Time."

15. Susan C. Gilchrist, Virginia J. Howard, Tomi Akinyemiju, et al., "Association of Sedentary Behavior with Cancer Mortality in Middle Aged and Older US Adults," *JAMA Oncology* 6, no. 8 (June 18, 2020), https://doi.org/10.1001/jamaoncol .2020.2045.

16. Hidde P. van der Ploeg, Tien Chey, Rosemary J. Korda, et al., "Sitting Time and All-Cause Mortality Risk in 222,497 Australian Adults," *Arch Internal Medicine* 172, no. 6 (2012), https://doi.org/10.1001/archinternmed.2011.2174.

17. Jared M. Tucker, Gregory J. Welk, and Nicholas K. Beyler, "Physical Activity in U.S. Adults: Compliance with the Physical Activity Guidelines for Americans," *American Journal of Preventative Medicine* 40, no. 4 (2011), https://doi.org/10.1016/j .amepre.2010.12.016.

18. James A. Levine, "Non-Exercise Activity Thermogenesis (NEAT)," *Best Practice and Research Clinical Endocrinology and Metabolism* 16, no. 4 (2002), https://doi .org/10.1053/beem.2002.0227.

19. Levine, "Non-Exercise Activity Thermogenesis (NEAT)."

20. Alia J. Crum and Ellen J. Langer, "Mind-set Matters: Exercise and the Placebo Effect," *Psychological Science* 18, no. 2 (2007), https://pubmed.ncbi.nlm.nih .gov/17425538/.

21. Laura Nauha, Heidi Jurvelin, Leena Ala-Mursula, et al., "Chronotypes and Objectively Measured Physical Activity and Sedentary Time at Midlife," *Scandinavian Journal of Medicine and Science in Sports* 30, no. 10 (2020), https://doi.org/10.1111 /sms.13753.

22. Marily Oppezzo and Daniel L. Schwartz, "Give Your Ideas Some Legs: The Positive Effect of Walking on Creative Thinking," *Journal of Experimental Psychology: Learning, Memory, and Cognition* 40, no. 4 (2014), https://www.apa.org/pubs /journals/releases/xlm-a0036577.pdf.

23. Philippa Margaret Dall, Sarah Lesley Hellen Ellis, Brian Martin Ellis, et al., "The Influence of Dog Ownership on Objective Measures of Free-Living Physical Activity and Sedentary Behavior in Community-Dwelling Older Adults: A Longitudinal Case-Controlled Study," *BMC Public Health* 17, no. 496 (2017), https://bmcpublichealth.biomedcentral.com/articles/10.1186/s12889-017-4422-5.

24. Carri Westgarth, Robert M. Christley, Christopher Jewell, et al., "Dog Owners Are More Likely to Meet Physical Activity Guidelines Than People Without a Dog: An Investigation of the Association Between Dog Ownership and Physical Activity Levels in a UK Community," *Scientific Reports* 9, no. 5704 (2019), https://www.nature.com/articles/s41598-019-41254-6.

25. Ann Regina Lurati, "Health Issues and Injury Risks with Prolonged Sitting and Sedentary Lifestyles," *Workplace Health and Safety* 66, no. 6 (2018), https://doi.org/10.1177/2165079917737558.

26. Brittany T. MacEwen, Dany J. MacDonald, and Jamie F. Burr, "A Systematic Review of Standing Treadmill Desks in the Workplace," *Preventative Medicine* 70 (2015), https://doi.org/10.1016/j.ypmed.2014.11.011.

27. MacEwen et al., "A Systematic Review of Standing Treadmill Desks in the Workplace."

28. Esther Gokhale and Socrates Adams, *8 Steps to a Pain-Free Back: Natural Posture Solutions for Pain in the Back, Neck, Shoulder, Hip, Knee, and Foot* (Lotus Publishing, 2013).

29. Ruth R. Sapsford, Carolyn A. Richardson, Christopher F. Maher, and Paul W. Hodges, "Pelvic Floor Muscle Activity in Different Sitting Postures in Continent and Incontinent Women," *Archives of Physical Medicine and Rehabilitation* 89, no. 9 (2008), https://doi.org/10.1016/j.apmr.2008.01.029.

30. Nicholas A. Levine and Brandon R. Rigby, "Thoracic Outlet Syndrome: Biomechanical and Exercise Considerations," *Healthcare* 6, no. 2 (2018), https://doi.org/10.3390/healthcare6020068.

31. Rudd Hortensius, Jack van Honk, Beatrice de Gelder, and David Terburg, "Trait Dominance Promotes Reflexive Staring at Masked Angry Body Postures," *PLOS One* 9, no. 12 (2014), https://doi.org/10.1371/journal.pone.0116232.

32. Rabeb Laatar, Hiba Kachouri, Rihab Borji, et al., "The Effect of Cell Phone Use on Postural Balance and Mobility in Older Compared to Young Adults," *Physiology and Behavior* 173, no. 1 (2017), https://doi.org/10.1016/j.physbeh.2017.02.031.

33. Xiaofei Guan, Guoxin Fan, Xinbo Wu, et al., "Photographic Measurement of Head and Cervical Posture When Viewing Mobile Phone: A Pilot Study," *European Spine Journal* 24 (2015), https://doi.org/10.1007/s00586-015-4143-3.

34. "Why Posture Matters," Harvard Health Publishing, 2017, https://www.health.harvard.edu/staying-healthy/why-good-posture-matters.

35. "The Egoscue Method," https://www.egoscue.com/what-is-egoscue/.

36. "What Is Posture Alignment Therapy?" Vital Balance Massage, http://www.vital balancetherapy.com/posture-alignment-therapy.

37. "What Is Posture Alignment Therapy?"

## Chapter 5: Biohacking Energy Through Exercise

1.  Raphael Bize, Jeffrey A. Johnson, and Ronald C. Plotnikoff, "Physical Activity Level and Health-Related Quality of Life in the General Adult Population: A Systematic Review," *Preventative Medicine* 45, no. 6 (2007), https://doi.org/10.1016/j .ypmed.2007.07.017.

2.  Sang-Ho Oh, Don-Kyu Kim, Shi-Uk Lee, Se Hee Jung, and Sang Yoon Lee, "Association Between Exercise Type and Quality of Life in a Community-Dwelling Older People: A Cross-Sectional Study," *PLOS One* 12, no. 12 (2017), https://doi .org/10.1371/journal.pone.0188335.

3.  Diane L. Gill, Cara C. Hammond, Erin J. Reifsteck, et al., "Physical Activity and Quality of Life," *Journal of Preventative Medicine and Public Health* 46, no. 1 (2013), https://dx.doi.org/10.3961%2Fjpmph.2013.46.S.S28.

4.  David A. Raichlen and Gene E. Alexander, "Adaptive Capacity: An Evolutionary Neuroscience Model Linking Exercise, Cognition, and Brain Health," *Trends in Neurosciences* 40, no. 7 (2017), https://doi.org/10.1016%2Fj.tins.2017.05.001.

5.  Alexandre Rebelo-Marques, Adriana De Sousa Lages, Renato Andrade, et al., "Aging Hallmarks: The Benefits of Physical Exercise," *Frontiers in Endocrinology* 9, no. 258 (2018), https://dx.doi.org/10.3389%2Ffendo.2018.00258.

6.  "Brain-Derived Neurotrophic Factor Controls Mitochondrial Transport in Neurons," *Journal of Biological Chemistry* 289, no. 3 (2014), https://www.ncbi.nlm.nih .gov/pmc/articles/PMC3894309/.

7.  Alejandro Santos-Lozano, Helios Paareja-Galeano, Fabian Sanchis-Gomar, et al., "Physical Activity and Alzheimer Disease: A Protective Association," *Mayo Clinic Proceedings* 91, no. 8 (2016), https://doi.org/10.1016/j.mayocp.2016.04.024.

8.  J. J. Steventon, C. Foster, H. Furby, D. Helme, et al., "Hippocampal Blood Flow Is increased After 20 Min of Moderate-Intensity Exercise," *Cerebral Cortex* 30, no. 2 (2020), https://doi.org/10.1093/cercor/bhz104.

9.  Valentina Perosa, Anastasia Priester, Gabriel Ziegler, et al., "Hippocampal Vascular Reserve Associated with Cognitive Performance and Hippocampal Volume," *Brain* 143, no. 2 (2020), https://doi.org/10.1093/brain/awz383.

10. Booth et al., "Role of Inactivity in Chronic Diseases."

11. Y. H. Wei, Y. S. Ma, H. C. Lee, C. F. Lee, C. Y. Lu, "Mitochondrial Theory of Aging Matures: Roles of mtDNA Mutation and Oxidative Stress in Human

Aging," *National Library of Medicine* 64, no. 5 (2001), https://pubmed.ncbi.nlm.nih.gov/11499335/.

12. Adeel Safdar, Jacqueline M. Bourgeois, Daniel I. Ogborn, and Mark A. Tarnopolsky, "Endurance Exercise Rescues Progeroid Aging and Induces Systemic Mitochondrial Rejuvenation in mtDNA Mutator Mice," *Biological Sciences* 108, no. 10 (2011), https://doi.org/10.1073/pnas.1019581108.

13. Bhupendra Singh, Trenton R. Schoeb, Prachi Bajpai, Andrzej Slominski, and Keshav K. Singh, "Reversing Wrinkled Skin and Hair Loss in Mice by Restoring Mitochondrial Function," *Cell Death and Disease* 9 (2018), https://www.nature.com/articles/s41419-018-0765-9.

14. Hannah Arem, Steven C. Moore, Alpa Patel, et al., "Leisure Time Physical Activity and Mortality: A Detailed Pooled Analysis of the Dose-Response Relationship," *JAMA Internal Medicine* 175, no. 6 (2015), https://doi.org/10.1001/jamainternmed.2015.0533.

15. U.S. Department of Health and Human Services, 2018 Physical Activity Guidelines for Americans, 2nd edition, https://health.gov/our-work/nutrition-physical-activity/physical-activity-guidelines/current-guidelines.

16. Arem et al., "Leisure Time Physical Activity and Mortality."

17. Barry A. Franklin, Paul D. Thompson, Salah S. al-Zaiti, et al., "Exercise-Related Acute Cardiovascular Events and Potential Deleterious Adaptations Following Long-Term Exercise Training: Placing the Risks into Perspective—An Update: A Scientific Statement from the American Heart Association," *Circulation* 141, no. 13 (2020), https://doi.org/10.1161/cir.0000000000000749.

18. James H. O'Keefe, Evan L. O'Keefe, and Carl J. Lavie, "The Goldilocks Zone for Exercise: Not Too Little, Not Too Much," *Missouri Medicine* 115, no. 2 (2018), https://pubmed.ncbi.nlm.nih.gov/30228692/.

19. "Million Women Study," National Cancer Institute, accessed June 14, 2022, https://epi.grants.cancer.gov/cohort-consortium/members/million-women-study.html.

20. O'Keefe et al., "The Goldilocks Zone for Exercise."

21. Thijs M. H. Eijsvogels, Paul D. Thompson, and Barry D. Franklin, "The 'Extreme Exercise Hypothesis': Recent Findings and Cardiovascular Health Implications," *Current Treatment Options in Cardiovascular Medicine* 20 (2018), https://dx.doi.org/10.1007%2Fs11936-018-0674-3.

22. Magnus Thorsten Jensen, Pouk Suadicani, Hans Oletlein, and Finn Gyntelberg, "Elevated Resting Heart Rate, Physical Fitness and All-Cause Mortality: A 16-Year Follow-up in the Copenhagen Male Study," *Heart* 99, no. 12 (2013), https://heart.bmj.com/content/99/12/882.full?sid=90e3623c-1250-4b94-928c-0a8f95c5b36b.

23. Mayo Clinic Staff, "Exercise Intensity: How to Measure It," Mayo Clinic, 2021, https://www.mayoclinic.org/healthy-lifestyle/fitness/in-depth/exercise-intensity/art-20046887.

24. Geetha Raghuveer, Jacob Hartz, David R. Lubans, et al., "Cardiorespiratory Fitness in Youth: An Important Marker of Health—A Scientific Statement from the American Heart Association," *Circulation* 142, no. 7 (2020), https://doi.org/10.1161/CIR.0000000000000866.

25. Booth et al., "Role of Inactivity in Chronic Diseases."

26. Zhihui Le, Jean Woo, and Timothy Kwok, "The Effect of Physical Activity and Cardiorespiratory Fitness on All-Cause Mortality in Hong Kong Chinese Older Adults," *Journals of Gerontology: Series A* 73, no. 8 (2018), https://doi.org/10.1093/gerona/glx180.

27. Katya Vargas-Oritz, Victoriano Perez-Vazquez, and Maciste H. Macias-Cervantes, "Exercise and Sirtuins: A Way to Mitochondrial Health in Skeletal Muscle," *International Journal of Molecular Sciences* 20, no. 11 (2019), https://doi.org/10.3390/ijms20112717.

28. Mikael Flockhart, Lina C. Nilsson, Senna Tais, et al., "Excessive Exercise Training Causes Mitochondrial Functional Impairment and Decreases Glucose Tolerance in Healthy Volunteers," *Cell Metabolism* 33, no. 5 (2021), https://www.cell.com/cell-metabolism/pdf/S1550-4131(21)00102-9.pdf.

29. Brian Glancy, Lisa M. Hartnell, Daniela Malide, et al., "Mitochondrial Reticulum for Cellular Energy Distribution in Muscle," *Nature* 523 (2015), https://doi.org/10.1038/nature14614.

30. Andre Lacroix, Tibor Hortobagyi, Rainer Beurskens, and Urs Granacher, "Effects of Supervised vs. Unsupervised Training Programs on Balance and Muscle Strength in Older Adults: A Systematic Review and Meta-Analysis," *Sports Medicine* 47 (2017), https://doi.org/10.1007/s40279-017-0747-6.

31. Osama Hamdy and Edward S. Horton, "Protein Content in Diabetes Nutrition Plan," *Current Diabetes Reports* 11, no. 2 (2011), https://doi.org/10.1007/s11892-010-0171-x.

32. Hamdy and Horton, "Protein Content in Diabetes Nutrition Plan."

33. Hiroyuki Kato, Katsuya Suzuki, Makoto Bannai, and Daniel R. Moore, "Protein Requirements Are Elevated in Endurance Athletes After Exercise as Determined by the Indicator Amino Acid Oxidation Method," *PLOS One* 11, no. 6 (2016), https://www.ncbi.nlm.nih.gov/pmc/articles/PMC4913918/.

34. "Optimal Protein Intake Guide," Examine, 2022, https://examine.com/guides/protein-intake/.

35. Tyler A. Churchward-Venne, Andrew M. Holwerda, Stuart M. Phillips, and Luc J. C. van Loon, "What Is the Optimal Amount of Protein to Support Post-Exercise

Skeletal Muscle Reconditioning in the Older Adult?" *Sports Medicine* 46, no. 9 (2016), https://pubmed.ncbi.nlm.nih.gov/26894275/.

36. Robert W. Morton, Kevin T. Murphy, Sean R. McKellar, et al., "A Systematic Review, Meta-analysis, and Meta-regression of the Effect of Protein Supplementation on Resistance Training–Induced Gains in Muscle Mass and Strength in Healthy Adults," *British Journal of Sports Medicine* 52, no. 6 (2018), https://doi.org/10.1136/bjsports-2017-097608.

37. David G. Le Couteur, Samantha M. Solon-Biet, Victoria C. Cogger, et al., "Branched Chain Amino Acids, Aging and Age-Related Health," *Ageing Res Rev.* (December 2020) 64:101198: 10.1016/j.arr.2020.101198.

38. Patricia de Paz-Lugo, Jose Antonio Lupianez, and Enrique Melendez-Hevia, "High Glycine Concentration Increases Collagen Synthesis by Articular Chondrocytes in Vitro: Acute Glycine Deficiency Could Be an Important Cause of Osteoarthritis," *Amino Acids* 50 (2018), https://doi.org/10.1007/s00726-018-2611-x.

39. Samuel McNerney, "A Brief Guide to Embodied Cognition: Why You Are Not Your Brain," *Scientific American,* November 4, 2011, https://blogs.scientificamerican.com /guest-blog/a-brief-guide-to-embodied-cognition-why-you-are-not-your-brain/.

40. Penelope Lein, George Picard, Joseph Baumgarden, and Roger Schneider, "Meditative Movement, Energetic, and Physical Analyses of Three Qigon Exercises: Unification of Eastern and Western Mechanistic Exercise Theory," *Medicines* 4, no. 4 (2017), https://dx.doi.org/10.3390%2Fmedicines4040069.

41. Lein et al., "Meditative Movement."

42. William James, *The Principles of Psychology* (Henry Holt and Company, 1890).

43. Rainer Kiss, Simon Schedler, and Thomas Muehlbauer, "Associations Between Types of Balance Performance in Healthy Individuals Across the Lifespan: A Systematic Review and Meta-Analysis," *Frontiers in Physiology* (2018), https://dx.doi.org/10.3389%2Ffphys.2018.01366.

44. Boguslaw Lipinski, "Biological Significance of Piezoelectricity in Relation to Acupuncture, Hatha Yoga, Osteopathic Medicine and Action of Air Ions," *Medical Hypotheses* 3, no. 1 (1977), https://doi.org/10.1016/0306-9877(77)90045-7.

45. Lipinski, "Biological Significance of Piezoelectricity."

46. Elizabeth Fain and Cara Weatherford, "Comparative Study of Millennials' (Age 20–34 Years) Grip and Lateral Pinch with the Norms," *Journal of Hand Therapy* 29, no. 4 (2016), https://doi.org/10.1016/j.jht.2015.12.006.

47. "Stu Phillips Discusses the Importance of Dietary Protein and Its Role in Muscle," *STEM-Talk* podcast, episode 82, February 25, 2019, https://www.ihmc.us/stem talk/episode-82/.

48. Shamini Ganasarajah, Sundstrom Poromaa, et al., "Objective Measures of Phys-

ical Performance Associated with Depression and/or Anxiety in Midlife Singaporean Women," *Menopause* 26, no. 9 (2019), https://doi.org/10.1097/gme.0000 000000001355.

49. Jarlo Ilano, "Badass for Life: Learn to Overcome the Challenges of Aging," GMB, 2020, https://gmb.io/badass-for-life/.

50. Manal A. Naseeb and Stella L. Volpe, "Protein and Exercise in the Prevention of Sarcopenia and Aging," *Nutrition Research* 40 (2017), https://doi.org/10.1016/j .nutres.2017.01.001.

51. Nuria Garatachea, Helios Pareja-Galeano, Fabian Sanchis-Gomar, et al., "Exercise Attenuates the Major Hallmarks of Aging," *Rejuvenation Research* 18, no. 1 (2015), https://doi.org/10.1089/rej.2014.1623.

52. Karen L. Troy, Megan E. Macuso, Tiffiny A. Butler, and Joshua E. Johnson, "Exercise Early and Often: Effects of Physical Activity and Exercise on Women's Bone Health," *International Journal of Environmental Research and Public Health* 15, no. 5 (2018), https://dx.doi.org/10.3390%2Fijerph15050878.

53. Amelia Guadalupe-Grau, Teresa Fuentes, Borja Guerra, and Jose A. L. Calbert, "Exercise and Bone Mass in Adults," *Sports Medicine* 39, no. 6 (2009), https:// pubmed.ncbi.nlm.nih.gov/19453205/.

## Chapter 6: Transforming Food into Energy

1. Ellen A. Wartella, Alice H. Lichtenstein, and Caitlin S. Boon, "Institute of Medicine (US) Committee on Examination of Front-of-Package Nutrition Rating Systems and Symbols," *Overview of Health and Diet in America. Front-of-Package Nutrition Rating Systems and Symbols: Phase I Report.* National Academies Press (US), 2010, 4, https://www.ncbi.nlm.nih.gov/books/NBK209844/; R Micha, JL Peñalvo, F Cudhea, et al., "Association Between Dietary Factors and Mortality from Heart Disease, Stroke, and Type 2 Diabetes in the United States," *JAMA* 317, no. 9 (March 2017): 912–924, doi:10.1001/jama.2017.0947.

2. Hyun Ah Park, "Fruit Intake to Prevent and Control Hypertension and Disease," *Korean Journal of Family Medicine* 42, no. 1 (2013), https://dx.doi.org /10.4082%2Fkjfm.20.0225.

3. Wartella et al., "Institute of Medicine (US) Committee on Examination of Front-of-Package Nutrition Rating Systems and Symbols"; "A Systematic Review of the Effects of Polyols on Gastrointestinal Health and Irritable Bowel Syndrome." *Advances in Nutrition* 2017, https://doi.org/10.3945/an.117.015560; James J. DiNicolantonio and James H. O'Keefe, "The Benefits of Omega-3 Fats for Stabilizing and Remodeling Atherosclerosis." *Missouri Medicine* 117, no. 1 (2020): 65–69.

4.  Mohammad Perwaiz Iqbal, "Trans Fatty Acids—A Risk Factor for Cardiovascular Disease," *Pakistan Journal of Medical Sciences* 30, no. 1 (2014), https://dx.doi.org/10.12669%2Fpjms.301.4525.

5.  "Artificial Trans Fats Banned in U.S.," Harvard School of Public Health, 2018, https://www.hsph.harvard.edu/news/hsph-in-the-news/us-bans-artificial-trans-fats/.

6.  Jeff Nobbs, "Is Oatly Oat Milk Healthy?," JeffNobbs.com, January 16, 2020, https://www.jeffnobbs.com/posts/is-oatly-healthy.

7.  Pew Research Center, "What's on Your Table? How America's Diet Has Changed over the Decades" https://www.pewresearch.org/fact-tank/2016/12/13/whats-on-your-table-how-americas-diet-has-changed-over-the-decades/.

8.  "Monounsaturated Fat," American Heart Association, June 1, 2015, https://www.heart.org/en/healthy-living/healthy-eating/eat-smart/fats/monounsaturated-fats.

9.  Marta Guasch-Ferre, Vanping Li, Walter L. Willett, et al., "Consumption of Olive Oil and Risk of Total and Cause-Specific Mortality Among U.S. Adults," *Journal of the American College of Cardiology* 79, no. 2 (2022), https://doi.org/10.1016/j.jacc.2021.10.041.

10. Mohammad G. Saklayen, "The Global Epidemic of the Metabolic Syndrome," *Current Hypertension Reports* 20, no. 2 (2018), https://www.ncbi.nlm.nih.gov/pmc/articles/PMC5866840/.

11. "Estimated Hypertension Prevalence, Treatment, and Control Among U.S. Adults," Million Hearts, 2021, https://millionhearts.hhs.gov/data-reports/hypertension-prevalence.html.

12. "Prevalence of Prediabetes Among Adults," Centers for Disease Control and Prevention, December 29, 2021, https://www.cdc.gov/diabetes/data/statistics-report/prevalence-of-prediabetes.html.

13. "Diabetes Statistics," Diabetes Research Institute Foundation, https://www.diabetesresearch.org/diabetes-statistics.

14. "Alzheimer's Disease Facts and Figures," Alzheimer's Association, https://www.alz.org/alzheimers-dementia/facts-figures.

15. "Heart Disease Facts," Centers for Disease Control and Prevention, https://www.cdc.gov/heartdisease/facts.htm.

16. Abdulaziz Malik, Amira Ramadan, Bhavya Vemuri, et al., "ω-3 Ethyl Ester Results in Better Cognitive Function at 12 and 30 Months Than Control in Cognitively Healthy Subjects with Coronary Artery Disease: A Secondary Analysis of a Randomized Clinical Trial," *American Journal of Clinical Nutrition* 113, no. 5 (2021), https://academic.oup.com/ajcn/article/113/5/1168/6155858?login=false.

17. James J. DiNicolantonio and James H. O'Keefe, "The Benefits of Omega-3 Fats

for Stabilizing and Remodeling Atherosclerosis," *Mo Med* 117, no. 1 (January–February 2020): 65–69. PMID: 32158053, PMCID: PMC7023944.

18. Tanya L. Blasbalg, Joseph R. Hibbeln, and Christopher E. Ramsden, et al., "Changes in Consumption of Omega-3 and Omega-6 Fatty Acids in the United States During the 20th Century," *American Journal of Clinical Nutrition* 93, no. 5 (2011), https://dx.doi.org/10.3945%2Fajcn.110.006643.

19. A. P. Simopoulous, "The Importance of the Ratio of Omega-6/Omega-3 Essential Fatty Acids," *Biomedicine and Pharmacotherapy* 56, no. 8 (2002), https://doi.org/10.1016/s0753-3322(02)00253-6.

20. Lucas F. R. Nascimento, Gabriela F. P. Souza, et al., "n-3 Fatty Acids Induce Neurogenesis of Predominantly POMC-Expression Cells in the Hypothalamus," *Diabetes* 65, no. 3 (2016), https://doi.org/10.2337/db15-0008.

21. Yang Hu, Frank B. Hu, and JoAnn E. Manson, "Marine Omega-3 Supplementation and Cardiovascular Disease: An Updated Meta-Analysis of 13 Randomized Controlled Trials Involving 127,477 Participants," *Journal of the American Heart Association* 8, no. 19 (2019), https://doi.org/10.1161/jaha.119.013543.

22. Nikos Stratakis, David V. Conti, Eva Borras, et al., "Association of Fish Consumption and Mercury Exposure During Pregnancy with Metabolic Health and Inflammatory Biomarkers in Children," *JAMA Network Open* 3, no. 3 (2020), https://dx.doi.org/10.1001%2Fjamanetworkopen.2020.1007.

23. Daniela Roxo de Souza, Bruno Luiz da Silva Pieri, Vitor Hugo Comim, et al., "Fish Oil Reduces Subclinical Inflammation, Insulin Resistance, and Atherogenic Factors in Overweight/Obese Type 2 Diabetes Mellitus Patients: A Pre-Post Pilot Study," *Journal of Diabetes and Its Complications* 34, no. 5 (2020), https://doi.org/10.1016/j.jdiacomp.2020.107553.

24. Beth McMurchie, Roberto King, Martin Lindley, et al., "Shedding Light on the Effect of Fish Oil Supplementation on Dark Adaptation Capabilities," *ChemRxiv* (2019), http://dx.doi.org/10.26434/chemrxiv.11302613.

25. Amanda M. Fretts, Jack L. Follis, Jennifer A. Nettleton, et al., "Consumption of Meat Is Associated with Higher Fasting Glucose and Insulin Concentrations Regardless of Glucose and Insulin Genetic Risk Scores: A Meta-Analysis of 50,345 Caucasians," *American Journal of Clinical Nutrition* 102, no. 5 (2015), https://dx.doi.org/10.3945%2Fajcn.114.101238.

26. Fretts et al., "Consumption of Meat Is Associated with Higher Fasting Glucose"; M. B. Schulze, J. E. Manson, W. C. Willett, and F. B. Hu, "Processed Meat Intake and Incidence of Type 2 Diabetes in Younger and Middle-Aged Women," *Diabetologia* 46 (2003), https://link.springer.com/content/pdf/10.1007/s00125-003-1220-7.pdf.

27. David E. Frankhouser, Sarah Steck, Michael G. Sovic, et al., "Dietary Omega-3 Fatty

Acid Intake Impacts Peripheral Blood DNA Methylation-Anti-Inflammatory Effects and Individual Variability in a Pilot Study." *Journal of Nutritional Biochemistry* 99 (January 1, 2022): 108839, https://doi.org/10.1016/j.jnutbio.2021.108839.

28. Carolina Donat-Vargas, Marika Berglund, Anders Glynn, et al., "Dietary Polychlorinated Biphenyls, Long-Chain n-3 Polyunsaturated Fatty Acids and Incidence of Malignant Melanoma," *European Journal of Cancer* 72 (February 1, 2017): 137–43, https://doi.org/10.1016/j.ejca.2016.11.016.

29. "Cheap Meat's Cost on Food Quality," Jefferson County Farmers and Neighbors, Inc., https://www.jfaniowa.org/real-cost-to-food-quality.

30. Evelyne Battaglia Richi, Beatrice Baumer, Beatrice Conrad, et al., "Health Risk Associated with Meat Consumption: A Review of Epidemiological Studies," *Vitamin and Nutrition Research* 85, no. 2 (2015), https://doi.org/10.1024/0300-9831/a000224.

31. H. D. Karsten, P. H. Patterson, R. Stout, and G. Crews, "Vitamins A, E and Fatty Acid Composition of the Eggs of Caged Hens and Pastured Hens," *Renewable Agriculture and Food Systems* 25, no. 1 (2010), http://dx.doi.org/10.1017/S1742170509990214.

32. "Essential Nutrient May Help Fight Alzheimer's Across Generations," ScienceDaily, 2019, https://www.sciencedaily.com/releases/2019/01/190108084424.htm.

33. Nicholas R. Fuller, Amanda Sainsbury, Ian D. Caterson, and Tania P. Markovic, "Egg Consumption and Human Cardio-Metabolic Health in People with and Without Diabetes," *Nutrients* 7, no. 9 (2015), https://dx.doi.org/10.3390%2Fnu7095344.

34. Edgar Antonio Reyes-Montano and Nohora Angelica Vega-Castro, "Plant Lectins with Insecticidal and Insectistatic Activities," in *Insecticides*, ed. Ghousia Begum (IntechOpen, 2017), https://www.intechopen.com/chapters/60115.

35. Z. X. Tan, R. Lal, and K. D. Wiebe, "Global Soil Nutrient Depletion and Yield Reduction," *Journal of Sustainable Agriculture* 26, no. 1 (2005), https://doi.org/10.1300/J064v26n01_10.

36. Shawn M. Wilder, David G. Le Couteur, and Stephen J. Simpson. "Diet Mediates the Relationship Between Longevity and Reproduction in Mammals," *Age* 35, no. 3 (2013), https://www.ncbi.nlm.nih.gov/pmc/articles/PMC3636383/.

37. Andrea Zuniga, Richard J. Stevenson, Mehmut K. Mahmut, and Ian D. Stephenson, "Diet Quality and the Attractiveness of Male Body Odor," *Evolution and Human Behavior* 38, no. 1 (2017), https://doi.org/10.1016/j.evolhumbehav.2016.08.002.

## Chapter 7: Blood Sugar Is the Ultimate Energy Biomarker

1. Alexandra E. Butler, Juliette Janson, Susan Bonner-Weir, et al., "β-Cell Deficit and Increased β-Cell Apoptosis in Humans with Type 2 Diabetes," *Diabetes* 52, no. 1 (2003), https://doi.org/10.2337/diabetes.52.1.102.

2.  "Diabetes Basics," Centers for Disease Control and Prevention, https://www.cdc
    .gov/diabetes/basics/index.html.

3.  "The Surprising Truth About Prediabetes," Centers for Disease Control and Preven-
    tion, https://www.cdc.gov/diabetes/library/features/truth-about-prediabetes.html.

4.  Jennal L. Johnson, Daniel S. Duick, et al., "Identifying Prediabetes Using Fast-
    ing Insulin Levels," *Endocrine Practice* 16, no. 1 (2010), https://doi.org/10.4158
    /ep09031.or.

5.  David Spero, "Do You Know Your Insulin Level?," *Diabetes Self-Management*, No-
    vember 22, 2017, https://www.diabetesselfmanagement.com/blog/do-you-know
    -your-insulin-level/.

6.  Mark F. McCarty, "AMPK Activation—Protean Potential for Boosting Health
    Span," *AGE* 36 (2014), https://dx.doi.org/10.1007%2Fs11357-013-9595-y.

7.  Tomoo Kondo, Mikiya Kishi, Takashi Fushimi, et al., "Vinegar Intake Reduces
    Body Weight, Body Fat Mass, and Serum Triglyceride Levels in Obese Japanese
    Subjects," *Bioscience, Biotechnology, and Biochemistry* 73, no. 8 (2014), https://www
    .tandfonline.com/doi/pdf/10.1271/bbb.90231.

8.  Saeko Imai, Michiaki Fukui, and Shizuo Kajiyama, "Effect of Eating Vegetables
    Before Carbohydrates on Glucose Excursions in Patients with Type 2 Diabe-
    tes," *Journal of Clinical Biochemistry and Nutrition* 54, no. 1 (2014), https://dx.doi
    .org/10.3164%2Fjcbn.13-67.

9.  Kimiko Nishino, Masaru Sakurai, Yumie Takeshita, and Toshinari Takamura,
    "Consuming Carbohydrates After Meat or Vegetables Lowers Postprandial Excur-
    sions of Glucose and Insulin in Nondiabetic Subjects," *Journal of Nutritional Science
    and Vitaminology* 64, no. 5 (2018), https://doi.org/10.3177/jnsv.64.316.

10. Jun Yin, Huili Yang, and Jianping Ye, "Efficacy of Berberine in Patients with
    Type 2 Diabetes Mellitus," *Metabolism: Clinical and Experimental* 57, no. 5 (2008),
    https://dx.doi.org/10.1016%2Fj.metabol.2008.01.013.

11. Mario Ciampolini and Riccardo Bianchi, "Training to Estimate Blood Glucose
    and to Form Associations with Initial Hunger," *Nutrition & Metabolism* 3 (2006),
    https://doi.org/10.1186/1743-7075-3-42.

## Chapter 8: The Gut-Energy Connection

1.  Céline Gérard and Hubert Vidal, "Impact of Gut Microbiota on Host Glyce-
    mic Control," *Frontiers in Endocrinology* 10 (2019), https://dx.doi.org/10.3389%
    2Ffendo.2019.00029.

2.  David Zeevi, Tal Korem, Niv Zamora et al., "Personalized Nutrition by Predic-
    tion of Glycemic Responses," *Cell* 163, no. 5 (2015), https://doi.org/10.1016/j.cell
    .2015.11.001.

3.  Teresa Vezza, Zaida Abad-Jiménez, Miguel Marti-Cabrera, et al., "Microbiota-Mitochondria Inter-Talk: A Potential Therapeutic Strategy in Obesity and Type 2 Diabetes," *Antioxidants* 9, no. 9 (2020), https://www.ncbi.nlm.nih.gov/pmc/articles/PMC7554719/.

4.  Vezza et al., "Microbiota-Mitochondria Inter-Talk."

5.  Vezza et al., "Microbiota-Mitochondria Inter-Talk."

6.  Kassem Maki, Edward. C. Deehan, Jens Walter, and Fredrik Bäckhed, "The Impact of Dietary Fiber on Gut Microbiota in Host Health and Disease," *Cell Host & Microbe* 23, no. 6 (2018), https://doi.org/10.1016/j.chom.2018.05.012.

7.  Yasmine Belkaid and Timothy Hand, "Role of the Microbiota in Immunity and Inflammation," *Cell* 157, no. 1 (2014), https://www.ncbi.nlm.nih.gov/pmc/articles/PMC4056765/#!po=52.3256.

8.  Connie C. Qiu, Roberto Caricchio, and Stefania Gallucci, "Triggers of Autoimmunity: The Role of Bacterial Infections in the Extracellular Exposure of Lupus Nuclear Autoantigens," *Frontiers in Endocrinology* (2019), https://www.frontiersin.org/articles/10.3389/fimmu.2019.02608/full.

9.  David J. A. Jenkins, Cyril W. C. Kendall, David G. Popovich, et al., "Effect of a Very-High-Fiber Vegetable, Fruit, and Nut Diet on Serum Lipids and Colonic Function," *Metabolism: Clinical and Experimental* 50, no. 4 (2001), https://doi.org/10.1053/meta.2001.21037.

10. Alex E. Mohr, Ralf Jäger, Katie C. Carpenter, et al., "The Athletic Gut Microbiota," *Journal of the International Society of Sports Nutrition* 17 (2020), https://jissn.biomedcentral.com/articles/10.1186/s12970-020-00353-w.

11. "Beta-Glucaronidase; Stool," Doctor's Data Inc., https://www.doctorsdata.com/beta-glucuronidase-stool/.

12. David W. Kaufman, Judith P. Kelly, Gary C. Curhan, et al., "*Oxalobacter formigenes* May Reduce the Risk of Calcium Oxalate Kidney Stones," *Journal of the American Society of Nephrology* 19, no. 6 (2008), https://dx.doi.org/10.1681%2FASN.2007101058.

13. S. C. Noonan and G. P. Savage, "Oxalate Content of Foods and Its Effect on Humans," *Asia Pacific Journal of Clinical Nutrition* 8, no. 1 (1999), https://pubmed.ncbi.nlm.nih.gov/24393738/; G. P. Savage, M. J. S. Charrier, and L. Vanhanen, "Bioavailability of Soluble Oxalate from Tea and the Effect of Consuming Milk with the Tea," *European Journal of Clinical Nutrition* 57 (2003), https://doi.org/10.1038/sj.ejcn.1601572.

14. W. P. N. Ganga W. Pathirana, S. A. Paul Chubb, Melissa J. Gillett, and Samuel D. Vasikaran, "Faecal Calprotectin," *Clinical Biochemist Reviews* 39, no. 3 (2018), https://www.ncbi.nlm.nih.gov/pmc/articles/PMC6370282/.

## Chapter 9: Biohacking Energy Metabolism

1. Ashima K. Kant, "Eating Patterns of U.S. Adults: Meals, Snacks, and Time of Eating," *Physiology & Behavior* 193, part B (2018), https://doi.org/10.1016/j.phys beh.2018.03.022.

2. Mark P. Mattson, Keelin Moehl, Nathaniel Ghena, et al., "Intermittent Metabolic Switching, Neuroplasticity and Brain Health," *Nature Reviews Neuroscience* 19 (2018), https://doi.org/10.1038/nrn.2017.156.

3. Deborah M. Muoio, "Metabolic Inflexibility: When Mitochondrial Indecision Leads to Metabolic Gridlock," *Cell* 159, no. 6 (2014), https://dx.doi.org/10.1016%2Fj.cell.2014.11.034.

4. Jason Fung, "Women and Fasting—Part 10," The Fasting Method, https://blog.thefastingmethod.com/women-and-fasting-part-10.

5. Stephen D. Anton, Keelin Moehl, William T. Donahoo, et al., "Flipping the Metabolic Switch: Understanding and Applying the Health Benefits of Fasting," *Obesity* 26, no. 2 (2018), https://dx.doi.org/10.1002%2Foby.22065.

6. Carlos López-Otín, Lorenzo Galluzzi, José M. P. Freije, et al., "Metabolic Control of Longevity," *Cell* 166, no. 4 (2016), https://doi.org/10.1016/j.cell.2016.07.031.

7. Anton et al., "Flipping the Metabolic Switch."

8. Kris Gunnars, "10 Health Benefits of Low-Carb and Ketogenic Diets," Healthline, November 20, 2018, https://www.healthline.com/nutrition/10-benefits-of-low-carb-ketogenic-diets#TOC_TITLE_HDR_2.

9. Jennifer Abbasi, "Interest in the Ketogenic Diet Grows for Weight Loss and Type 2 Diabetes," *JAMA* 319, no. 3 (2018), https://doi.org/10.1001/jama.2017.20639.

10. Abbasi, "Interest in the Ketogenic Diet Grows."

11. Shubhroz Gill and Satchidananda Panda, "A Smartphone App Reveals Erratic Diurnal Eating Patterns in Humans That Can Be Modulated for Health Benefits," *Cell Metabolism* 22, no. 5 (2015), https://dx.doi.org/10.1016%2Fj.cmet.2015.09.005.

12. Yuan, Xiaojie, Jiping Wang, Shuo Yang, Mei Gao, Lingxia Cao, Xumei Li, Dongxu Hong, Suyan Tian, and Chenglin Sun. "Effect of Intermittent Fasting Diet on Glucose and Lipid Metabolism and Insulin Resistance in Patients with Impaired Glucose and Lipid Metabolism: A Systematic Review and Meta-Analysis." *International Journal of Endocrinology* 2022 (March 24, 2022): 6999907. https://doi.org/10.1155/2022/6999907.

13. Przemysław Domaszewski, Mariusz Konieczny, Paweł Pakosz, et al., "Effect of a Six-Week Intermittent Fasting Intervention Program on the Composition of the Human Body in Women over 60 Years of Age." *International Journal of*

*Environmental Research and Public Health* 17, no. 11, January 2020: 4138. https://doi.org/10.3390/ijerph17114138.

14. Yuriy P. Zverev, "Effects of Caloric Deprivation and Satiety on Sensitivity of the Gustatory System," *BMC Neuroscience* 5 (2004), https://dx.doi.org/10.1186%2F1471-2202-5-5.

## Chapter 10: Stress Drains Your Batteries

1. J. Douglas Bremner, "Stress and Brain Atrophy," *CNS and Neurological Disorders Drug Targets* 5, no. 5 (2006), https://www.ncbi.nlm.nih.gov/pmc/articles/PMC3269810/.

2. Mithu Storoni, *Stress-Proof: The Scientific Solution to Protect Your Brain and Body—and Be More Resilient Every Day* (TarcherPerigee, 2017).

3. Chris Hardy and Marty Gallagher, *Strong Medicine: How to Conquer Chronic Disease and Achieve Your Full Genetic Potential* (Dragon Door Publications, 2015).

4. Jos F. Brosschot, Bart Verkuil, and Julian F. Thayer, "Exposed to Events That Never Happen: Generalized Unsafety, the Default Stress Response, and Prolonged Autonomic Activity," *Neuroscience and Biobehavioral Reviews* 74, part B (2017), https://doi.org/10.1016/j.neubiorev.2016.07.019.

5. Brosschot et al., "Exposed to Events That Never Happen."

6. Brosschot et al., "Exposed to Events That Never Happen."

7. Allana T. Forde, Mario Sims, Paul Muntner, et al., "Discrimination and Hypertension Risk Among African Americans in the Jackson Heart Study," *Hypertension* 76, no. 3 (2020), https://doi.org/10.1161/HYPERTENSIONAHA.119.14492.

8. Gary Housley and Marion Burgess, "Health Effects of Environmental Noise Pollution," Australian Academy of Science, November 21, 2017, https://www.science.org.au/curious/earth-environment/health-effects-environmental-noise-pollution.

9. Brosschot et al., "Exposed to Events That Never Happen."

10. Pete McBride and Erik Weihenmayer, "Seeing Silence: One Photographer's Mission to Find the World's Quietest Places," NPR, October 3, 2021, https://www.npr.org/2021/10/03/1042831854/seeing-silence-one-photographers-mission-to-find-the-worlds-quietest-places.

11. Science Communication Unit, University of West England, "Noise Impacts on Health," European Commission Science for Environment Policy, January 2015, https://ec.europa.eu/environment/integration/research/newsalert/pdf/47si.pdf.

12. Qing Li, "Effect of Forest Bathing Trips on Human Immune Function," *Environmental Health and Preventative Medicine* 15 (2009), https://dx.doi.org/10.1007%2Fs12199-008-0068-3.

13. Leila Ben Amor, Natalie Grizenko, George Schwartz, et al., "Perinatal Complications in Children with Attention-Deficit Hyperactivity Disorder and Their Unaffected Siblings," *Journal of Psychiatry and Neuroscience* 30, no. 2 (2005), https://www.ncbi.nlm.nih.gov/pmc/articles/PMC551167/; Kaiser Permanente, "ADHD Linked to Oxygen Deprivation Before Birth," ScienceDaily, December 10, 2012, https://www.sciencedaily.com/releases/2012/12/121210080833.htm.

14. "Fast Facts: Preventing Child Sexual Abuse," Centers for Disease Control and Prevention, April 6, 2022, https://www.cdc.gov/violenceprevention/childsexual abuse/fastfact.html.

15. Steven E. Mock and Susan M. Arai, "Childhood Trauma and Chronic Illness in Adulthood: Mental Health and Socioeconomic Status as Explanatory Factors and Buffers," *Frontiers in Psychology* 1 (2011), https://dx.doi.org/10.3389%2Ffps yg.2010.00246.

16. Mock and Arai, "Childhood Trauma and Chronic Illness in Adulthood."

17. Brosschot et al., "Exposed to Events That Never Happen."

18. Jane Stevens (PACEs Connection Staff). "What ACEs and PCEs Do You Have?" PACEs Connection, https://www.pacesconnection.com/blog/got-your -ace-resilience-scores.

19. Gay Hendricks, *The Big Leap: Conquer Your Hidden Fear and Take Life to the Next Level* (HarperOne, 2010).

20. Pete Walker, MA Psychotherapy, http://pete-walker.com/.

## Chapter 11: Biohacking to Recharge

1. If you'd like to take a test that does offer a score, you can find a widely used stress scale called the Holmes-Rahe Life Stress Inventory on my website.

2. H. R. Berthoud and W. L. Neuhuber, "Functional and Chemical Anatomy of the Afferent Vagal System," *Autonomic Neuroscience: Basic and Clinical 85* (2000), https://pubmed.ncbi.nlm.nih.gov/11189015/.

3. David Peters, "The Neurobiology of Resilience," *InnovAiT* 9, no. 6 (2016), https://doi.org/10.1177%2F1755738016641980.

4. Bangalore G. Kalyani, Ganesan Venkatasubramanian, Rashmi Arasappa, et al., "Neurohemodynamic Correlates of 'OM' Chanting: A Pilot Functional Magnetic Resonance Imaging Study," *International Journal of Yoga* 4, no. 1 (2011), https://doi .org/10.4103%2F0973-6131.78171.

5. Sengui Yaman-Sozbir, Sultan Ayaz-Alkaya, and Burcu Bayrak-Kahraman, "Effect of Chewing Gum on Stress, Anxiety, Depression, Self-Focused Attention, and Academic Success: A Randomized Controlled Study," *Stress and Health* 35, no. 4 (2019), https://doi.org/10.1002/smi.2872.

6. "Stress Management: Breathing Exercises for Relaxation," University of Michigan Health, August 31, 2020, https://www.uofmhealth.org/health-library/uz2255.

7. Nina E. Fultz, Giorgio Bonmassar, Kawin Setsonpop, et al., "Coupled Electrophysiological, Hemodynamic, and Cerebrospinal Fluid Oscillations in Human Sleep," *Science* 366, no. 6465 (2019), https://www.science.org/doi/10.1126/science .aax5440.

8. Daniel J. Levendowski, Charlene Gamaldo, Erik K. St. Louis, et al., "Head Position During Sleep: Potential Implications for Patients with Neurodegenerative Disease," *Journal of Alzheimer's Disease* 67, no. 2 (2019), https://dx.doi .org/10.3233%2FJAD-180697; Hedok Lee, Lulu Xie, Mei Yu, et al., "The Effect of Body Posture on Brain Glymphatic Transport," *Journal of Neuroscience* 35, no. 31 (2015), https://doi.org/10.1523/JNEUROSCI.1625-15.2015.

9. J. Kabat-Zinn, "Mindfulness-Based Interventions in Context: Past, Present, and Future," *Clinical Psychology: Science and Practice* 10, no. 2 (2003), https://psycnet .apa.org/doi/10.1093/clipsy.bpg016.

10. Carolyn Y. Fang, Diane K. Reibel, Margaret L. Longacre, et al., "Enhanced Psychosocial Well-Being Following Participation in a Mindfulness-Based Stress Reduction Program Is Associated with Increased Natural Killer Cell Activity," *Journal of Alternative and Complementary Medicine* 16, no. 5 (2010), https://doi.org /10.1089/acm.2009.0018.

11. Simon B. Goldberg, Raymond P. Tucker, Preston A. Greene, et al., "Mindfulness-Based Interventions for Psychiatric Disorders: A Systematic Review and Meta-Analysis," *Clinical Psychology Review* 59 (2018), https://dx.doi.org/10.1016%2Fj .cpr.2017.10.011.

12. Raphael Millière, Robin L. Carhart-Harris, Leor Roseman, et al., "Psychedelics, Meditation, and Self-Consciousness," *Frontiers in Psychology* 9 (2018), https://doi .org/10.3389/fpsyg.2018.01475.

13. Kristen Sparrow and Brenda Golianu, "Does Acupuncture Reduce Stress Over Time? A Clinical Heart Rate Variability Study in Hypertensive Patients," *Medical Acupuncture* 26, no. 5 (2014), https://www.ncbi.nlm.nih.gov/pmc/articles/PMC 4203477/.

14. Peta Stapleton, Gabrielle Crichton, Debbie Sabot, and Hayley Maree O'Neill, "Reexamining the Effect of Emotional Freedom Techniques on Stress Biochemistry: A Randomized Controlled Trial," *Psychological Trauma* 12, no. 8 (2020), https://pubmed.ncbi.nlm.nih.gov/32162958/.

15. Magdalena Błażek, Maria Kaźmierczak, and Tomasz Besta, "Sense of Purpose in Life and Escape from Self as the Predictors of Quality of Life in Clinical Samples," *Journal of Religion and Health* 54 (2015), https://doi.org/10.1007/s10943 -014-9833-3.

16. Aliya Alimujiang, Ashley Wiensch, Jonathan Boss, et al., "Association Between Life Purpose and Mortality Among US Adults Older Than 50 Years," *JAMA Network Open* 2, no. 5 (2019), https://doi.org/10.1001/jamanetworkopen.2019.4270.

17. "Dharma Inquiry," CivilizationEmerging.com, September 28, 2019, https://civilizationemerging.com/dharma-inquiry/.

18. Hielke Buddelmeyer and Nattavudh Powdthavee, "Can Having Internal Locus of Control Insure Against Negative Shocks? Psychological Evidence from Panel Data," *Journal of Economic Behavior & Organization* 122 (2016), https://doi.org/10.1016%2Fj.jebo.2015.11.014.

## Chapter 12: The Hormone-Energy Connection

1. Meg Walters, "Is There Really a Connection Between Your Menstrual Cycle and the Moon?," Healthline, August 31, 2021, https://www.healthline.com/health/womens-health/menstrual-cycle-and-the-moon.

2. Julie A. Hobart and Douglas R. Smucker, "The Female Athlete Triad," *American Family Physician* 61, no. 11 (2000), https://www.aafp.org/pubs/afp/issues/2000/0601/p3357.html.

3. "PCOS (Polycystic Ovary Syndrome) and Diabetes," Centers for Disease Control and Prevention, March 24, 2020, https://www.cdc.gov/diabetes/basics/pcos.html#.

4. Andrea Dunaif, "Insulin Resistance and the Polycystic Ovary Syndrome: Mechanism and Implications for Pathogenesis," *Endocrine Reviews* 18, no. 6 (1997), https://doi.org/10.1210/edrv.18.6.0318.

5. Nuzhat Shaikh, Roshan Dadachanji, and Srabani Mukherjee, "Genetic Markers of Polycystic Ovary Syndrome: Emphasis on Insulin Resistance," *International Journal of Medical Genetics* 2014 (2014), https://doi.org/10.1155/2014/478972.

6. Alida Iacobellis, "RED-S: The New and Improved Female Athlete Triad," SportsMD.com, June 12, 2019, https://www.sportsmd.com/2019/06/12/red-s-the-new-and-improved-female-athlete-triad/.

7. Jasmine A. McDonald, Abishek Goyal, and Mary Beth Terry, "Alcohol Intake and Breast Cancer Risk: Weighing the Overall Evidence," *Current Breast Cancer Reports* 5 (2013), https://doi.org/10.1007%2Fs12609-013-0114-z.

8. "Fasting Mimicking Program & Longevity," ValterLongo.com, https://www.valterlongo.com/fasting-mimicking-program-and-longevity/.

9. "Menopause," Mayo Clinic, https://www.mayoclinic.org/diseases-conditions/menopause/symptoms-causes/syc-20353397#.

## Chapter 13: Biohacking Your Sexual Spark

1. K. E. Sims, "Why Does Passion Wane? A Qualitative Study of Hypoactive Sexual Desire Disorder in Married Women," PhD dissertation, University of Nevada–Las Vegas, January 1, 2007, https://doi.org/10.25669/29J8-AQLO.

2. S. A. Kingsberg, "Attitudinal Survey of Women Living with Low Sexual Desire," *Journal of Women's Health* 23, no. 10 (2003), https://doi.org/10.1089/jwh.2014.4743.

3. Misia Landau, "Trans Fats May Raise Risk of Infertility," Harvard Medical School, February 9, 2007, https://hms.harvard.edu/news/trans-fats-may-raise-risk-infertility#.

4. Brooke V. Rossi, Katharine F. Berry, Mark D. Hornstein, et al., "Effect of Alcohol Consumption on In Vitro Fertilization," *Obstetrics & Gynecology* 117, no. 1 (2011), https://doi.org/10.1097%2FAOG.0b013e31820090e1.

5. B. Jacobsen, K. Jaceldo-Siegl, S. F. Knutsen, et al., "Soy Isoflavone Intake and the Likelihood of Ever Becoming a Mother: The Adventist Health Study-2," *International Journal of Women's Health* 6 (2014), http://dx.doi.org/10.2147/IJWH.S57137.

6. Lisa K. Brents, "Marijuana, the Endocannabinoid System and the Female Reproductive System," *Yale Journal of Biology and Medicine* 89, no. 2 (2016), https://pubmed.ncbi.nlm.nih.gov/27354844/.

7. S. L. Mumford, K. S. Flannagan, J. G. Radoc, et al., "Cannabis Use While Trying to Conceive: A Prospective Cohort Study Evaluating Associations with Fecundability, Live Birth and Pregnancy Loss," *Human Reproduction* 36, no. 5 (2021), https://doi.org/10.1093/humrep/deaa355.

## Chapter 14: Connection Is the Key to Longevity

1. Liz Mineo, "Good Genes Are Nice, but Joy Is Better," *Harvard Gazette,* April 11, 2017, https://news.harvard.edu/gazette/story/2017/04/over-nearly-80-years-harvard-study-has-been-showing-how-to-live-a-healthy-and-happy-life/; "Welcome to the Harvard Study of Adult Development," Harvard Second Generation Study, https://www.adultdevelopmentstudy.org/; R. J. Waldinger and M. S. Schultz, "What's Love Got to Do with It? Social Functioning, Perceived Health, and Daily Happiness in Married Octogenarians, *Psychology and Aging* 25, no. 2 (2010), https://doi.org/10.1037%2Fa0019087.

2. Martin Picard and Carmen Sandi, "The Social Nature of Mitochondria: Implications for Human Health," *Neuroscience & Biobehavioral Reviews* 120 (2021), https://doi.org/10.1016/j.neubiorev.2020.04.017.

3. Martin Picard, Aric A. Prather, Eli Puterman, et al., "A Mitochondrial Health Index Sensitive to Mood and Caregiving Stress," *Biological Psychiatry* 84, no. 1 (2018), https://doi.org/10.1016/j.biopsych.2018.01.012.

4.  Danielle L. Clark, Jean L. Raphael, and Amy L. McGuire, "HEADS: Social Media Screening in Adolescent Primary Care," *Pediatrics Perspectives* 141, no. 6 (2018), https://doi.org/10.1542/peds.2017-3655.

5.  J. M. Twenge, A. B. Cooper, T. E. Joiner, et al., "Age, Period, and Cohort Trends in Mood Disorder Indicators and Suicide-Related Outcomes in a Nationally Representative Dataset, 2005–2017," *Journal of Abnormal Psychology* 128, no. 3 (2019), https://doi.org/10.1037/abn0000410.

6.  Tony Durkee, Vladimir Carli, Birgitta Floderus, et al., "Pathological Internet Use and Risk-Behaviors Among European Adolescents," *International Journal of Environmental Research and Public Health* 13, no. 3 (2016), https://dx.doi.org/10.3390%2Fijerph13030294.

7.  Adam Gazzaley, "The Cognition Crisis: Anxiety. Depression. ADHD. The Human Brain Is in Trouble. Technology Is a Cause—and a Solution," *Elemental*, July 9, 2018, https://elemental.medium.com/the-cognition-crisis-a1482e889fcb.

8.  Jiyoung Park, Shinobu Kitayama, Mayumi Karasawa, et al., "Clarifying the Links Between Social Support and Health: Culture, Stress, and Neuroticism Matter," *Journal of Health Psychology* 18, no. 2 (2013), https://doi.org/10.1177%2F1359105312439731.

9.  Cheuk Yin Ho, "Better Health with More Friends: The Role of Social Capital in Producing Health," *Health Economics* 25, no. 1 (2016), https://doi.org/10.1002/hec.3131.

10.  Park et al., "Clarifying the Links Between Social Support and Health."

11.  John T. Cacioppo and Stephanie Cacioppo, "Social Relationships and Health: The Toxic Effects of Perceived Social Isolation," *Social and Personality Psychology Compass* 8, no. 2 (2014), https://doi.org/10.1111%2Fspc3.12087.

12.  Noralou P. Roos and Evelyn Shapiro, "The Manitoba Longitudinal Study on Aging: Preliminary Findings on Health Care Utilization by the Elderly," *Medical Care* 19, no. 6 (1981), https://doi.org/10.1097/00005650-198106000-00007.

13.  M. J. Heisel and P. R. Duberstein, "Suicide Prevention in Older Adults," *Clinical Psychology* 12, no. 3 (2005), https://psycnet.apa.org/doi/10.1093/clipsy.bpi030.

14.  Enrique Burunat, "Love Is Not an Emotion," *Psychology* 7, no. 14 (2016), https://doi.org/10.4236/psych.2016.714173.

15.  Daniel S. Quintana and Adam J. Guastella, "An Allostatic Theory of Oxytocin," *Trends in Cognitive Sciences* 24, no. 7 (2020), https://doi.org/10.1016/j.tics.2020.03.008.

16.  Soo Min Hong, Jeong-Kyung Ko, Jung-Joon Moon, and Youl-Ri Kim, "Oxytocin: A Potential Therapeutic for Obesity," *Journal of Obesity & Metabolic Syndrome* 30, no. 2 (2021), https://doi.org/10.7570/jomes20098.

17. Evan A. Bordt, Caroline J. Smith, Tyler G. Demarest, et al., "Mitochondria, Oxytocin, and Vasopressin: Unfolding the Inflammatory Protein Response," *Neurotoxicity Research* 36, no. 2 (2019), https://doi.org/10.1007/s12640-018-9962-7.

18. C. Sue Carter, William M. Kenkel, Evan L. MacLean, et al., "Is Oxytocin 'Nature's Medicine'?," *Pharmacological Reviews* 72, no. 4 (2020), https://pharmrev.aspet journals.org/content/72/4/829.

19. C. Sue Carter and Stephen W. Porges, "The Biochemistry of Love: An Oxytocin Hypothesis," *EMBO Reports* 14, no. 1 (2013), https://doi.org/10.1038/embor .2012.191.

20. D. W. Pfaff, *Drive: Neurobiological and Molecular Mechanisms of Sexual Motivation* (MIT Press, 1999).

21. S. M. Merrill, "An Exploration of the Transition from Romantic Infatuation to Adult Attachment," doctoral thesis, Cornell University, August 30, 2018, https:// doi.org/10.7298/X45M640Z.

22. Z. Zou, H. Song, Y. Zhang, and X. Zhang, "Romantic Love vs. Drug Addiction May Inspire a New Treatment for Addiction," *Frontiers in Psychology* 7 (2016), https://doi.org/10.3389/fpsyg.2016.01436.

23. G. J. O. Fletcher, J. A. Simpson, L. Campbell, and N. C. Overall, "Pair-Bonding, Romantic Love, and Evolution: The Curious Case of *Homo sapiens*," *Perspectives on Psychological Science* 10, no. 1 (2015), https://doi.org/10.1177/1745691614561683.

# Index

# About the Author

**Molly Maloof, MD,** provides health optimization and personalized medicine to high-achieving entrepreneurs, investors, and technology executives. She taught a pioneering course on healthspan in the Wellness Department of the Stanford University School of Medicine for three years before launching her own company, inspired by her unique philosophy of health. Since 2012, she has worked as an adviser or consultant to more than fifty companies in the digital health, consumer health, and biotechnology industries. Dr. Maloof is on the frontier of personalized medicine, digital-health technologies, biofeedback-assisted lifestyle interventions, psychedelic medicine, and science-backed wellness products and services.